Praise for Dr. Mayer Eisenstein

CW00709170

Make an Informed V

"This is an excellent book, which I will ⟨
I believe it is the best single volume on the su⌐y
Eisenstein and Neil Miller deserve our gratitude, first, for the thoroughness of their research, which includes peer-reviewed journal studies, official vaccine adverse event reports (VAERS), firsthand accounts by parents, and concise, easy-to-read summaries of their own. Second, for their sober, balanced, and thoughtful tone—for resisting the temptation to say that all vaccines are bad under all circumstances and should never be given. The message of this book is that there is a serious downside to vaccines being mandated for everyone, which is seldom acknowledged or taken seriously, and that the obvious solution is simply to make them optional, as has long been the case in other developed countries, rather than a sacrament of modern medicine, as they are here in the United States." —*Richard Moskowitz, MD, Family Medicine*

"*Make an Informed Vaccine Decision* is an absolute MUST READ for medical professionals, especially pediatricians, as well as for motivated laypeople seeking facts and proper guidance, not more political policy masquerading as scientific truth." —*Thomas E. Levy, MD, JD, Cardiology and Internal Medicine*

"*Make an Informed Vaccine Decision* should be REQUIRED READING for all medical students, physicians, nurses, clinic managers, and medical school professors, not to mention all parents and policymakers. As a medical doctor, I learned a lot from this book and wholeheartedly recommend it to both professionals and laypeople. It is well researched with extensive references. In addition, knowing that Dr. Eisenstein has NO cases of autism in his unvaccinated patients is quite revealing. His forward-thinking medical practice has been a great gift to the thousands of children and their parents that he has served. Thank you, Dr. Eisenstein, for your courage in practicing compassionate, patient-centered medicine all these years and now teaching the rest of us how important it is to actually take seriously the Hippocratic Oath." —*Gary G. Kohls, MD, Family Medicine*

"This book is a MUST READ for anyone considering vaccination. Dr. Eisenstein brilliantly provides the reader with a realistic picture of potential benefits as well as possible consequences of each vaccine in a non-biased approach. Well supported by cited medical literature, parents will be prepared to make truly informed decisions that can affect their children for generations to come."
—*Jerry Kartzinel, MD, FAAP, Board Certified Pediatrics*

"As a mother and holistic pediatrician, I chose to stop vaccinating my children. As a traditionally-trained medical doctor, I was taught to educate parents and patients that vaccine benefits outweigh their risks. After I became a parent, I realized immunizations are not safe for everyone and that physicians have no way to screen children for vaccine safety. Since I am uncertain if vaccines will do more harm than good, I now advise parents and patients to make informed decisions *before* vaccinating their children or themselves. *Make an Informed Vaccine Decision* is a comprehensive research-based review for parents wanting to hear the untold story about vaccines. Thank you for this reputable resource; I will continually recommend this book to parents and healthcare professionals alike." —*Susan McCreadie, MD, Board Certified Pediatrician; Director of Pediatric Holistic Medicine and NourishMD.com*

"Make an Informed Vaccine Decision by Dr. Mayer Eisenstein offers a rigorous scientific discussion showing that many vaccinations have poor benefit-to-risk ratios, sometimes causing life-threatening disorders. As a medical doctor and scientist, this book has increased my awareness of the research confirming unacceptable health risks and questionable benefit outcomes of most vaccines. As a Rabbi, I am appalled at the moral bankruptcy of the vaccine manufacturers in collaboration with government agencies who have violated six of the Ten Commandments with their deliberately false, misleading, or 'doctored' information, apparently to increase profits. In my role as a grandfather, I am alarmed and concerned for my grandchildren, and for all children, at the mindless risks they are exposed to in current vaccination campaigns. This book is a MUST READ for all parents and grandparents."

—Rabbi Gabriel Cousens, MD, MD(H), Diplomat American Board of Holistic Medicine; Director of the Tree of Life Rejuvenation Center

"Make an Informed Vaccine Decision is a prodigiously researched book. It is also the most honest, comprehensive, and informative book ever written on this troubling topic. It contains facts that others want hidden, a perfect antidote to official propaganda. Read it and then read it again. The information it contains will save lives. Dr. Eisenstein has delivered a pearl of a book, and with it has become a worthy successor to the late, well-respected vaccine iconoclast, Dr. Robert Mendelsohn. This book should be REQUIRED READING for all new parents—and for all medical students—before they are indoctrinated into a dubious vaccine agenda." *—Keith Scott-Mumby, MD, MB ChB, PhD*

"Dr. Mayer Eisenstein impartially weighs the pros and cons of vaccines. He encourages readers to study the information so that they can make informed vaccine decisions. This is an excellent resource, especially for American families."
—Donald W. Miller, Jr., MD, Professor of Cardiac Surgery, University of Washington School of Medicine

"Make an Informed Vaccine Decision by Dr. Mayer Eisenstein is a credible and thorough guide for parents who are concerned about the safety and efficacy of our current vaccination schedule. Drawing from the medical literature, peer-reviewed journals, and personal experience, Dr. Eisenstein takes a hard look at vaccines—as well as the politics and business behind the industry—and is not afraid to question the prevailing pro-vaccination perspective. The best healthcare and parenting choices are always informed and educated decisions. Dr. Eisenstein's powerful book empowers parents through knowledge, giving them the opportunity to be the best advocates for their children, as they should be."
—Nancy Massotto, PhD, Executive Director, Holistic Moms Network

In *Make an Informed Vaccine Decision,* Dr. Mayer Eisenstein has done an excellent review of each infection which the vaccines address, and he has shown clear evidence that they can create permanent disabilities and even death. His personal experience with thousands of children who were not vaccinated, without a single case of autism, has dramatic implications. Holistic medical doctors—a disregarded minority—concur with Dr. Eisenstein about the harmful effects of the multitude of administered vaccines. I am sure that his mentor, Dr. Robert Mendelsohn, would be proud of his pupil and very pleased with this publication.
—Abram Ber, MD, Homeopathic and Holistic Physician

Make an Informed Vaccine Decision

For the Health of Your Child

A Parent's Guide
to Childhood Shots

Mayer Eisenstein, MD, JD, MPH

with Neil Z. Miller

New Atlantean Press
Santa Fe, New Mexico

Make an Informed Vaccine Decision

For the Health of Your Child

A Parent's Guide
to Childhood Shots

ISBN: 978-188121736-7

Library of Congress Cataloging-in-Publication Data

Eisenstein, Mayer, 1946-
  Make an informed vaccine decision for the health of your child : a parent's guide to childhood shots / by Mayer Eisenstein and Neil Z. Miller.
    p. cm.
  Includes bibliographical references and index.
  ISBN 978-1-881217-36-7
  1. Vaccination of children—Popular works. I. Miller, Neil Z. II. Title.
  RJ240.E37 2010
  614.4'7083—dc22
                        2009041520

Printed in the United States of America

Published by:
New Atlantean Press
PO Box 9638
Santa Fe, NM 87504
www.new-atlantean.com

*This publication is dedicated
to parents and their children.*

Warning/Disclaimer/Disclosure

Contents

8 Make an Informed Vaccine Decision

Introduction

In 1968, I began my medical education at the University of Illinois Medical School. The first two years are straight book learning: anatomy, physiology, biochemistry. In the second two years you go through a rotation of pediatrics, internal medicine, and surgery. In 1970, as a third-year medical student, I took a class on pediatrics where I first met Dr. Robert Mendelsohn, who was my professor. We developed a lifelong relationship: he attended the birth of my first child and became the godfather to my six children.

Dr. Mendelsohn was beyond brilliant, and had a profound influence on my health philosophy. He was the national medical director of Project Head Start (appointed to this post by President Lyndon B. Johnson), chairman of the Medical Licensure Committee for the state of Illinois, and a director of Chicago's Michael Reese Hospital. Dr. Mendelsohn was a distinguished doctor in every respect...*but he did not believe in vaccines!* He also warned parents to be wary of allopathic medicine. By 1973, he was convinced that "every vaccine causes neurological damage."

When I graduated from medical school I started working with Dr. Mendelsohn. I also opened up my own practice, Homefirst® Health Services. Dr. Mendelsohn was still under a Head Start contract in Chicago and I worked at his clinic for a day or two a week while I was also delivering babies at home. I delivered more babies at County in the six months while I was there than most doctors deliver in a lifetime. The homebirth business started growing, and in 1974 I opened an office on the north side of Chicago. I gave every family the choice to vaccinate or not. That started from the first day I was in practice, and it wasn't something I pushed.

A few years later, I attended the University of Wisconsin Medical School and graduated with a Masters degree in Public Health (MPH). The program consisted of courses in infectious disease, bio-statistics, epidemiology, and vaccination. As a *private* practicing physician, you apply the knowledge that you gained in medical school to your individual patients hoping to make your families healthier. As a *public* health doctor you look at a population and consider measures that can make a group of people healthier. So, the second degree that I have is a Masters of Public Health and I am Board certified in Preventive Medicine. The World Health Organization (WHO) is essentially made up of doctors of Public Health. It means that you have extra training and expertise in looking at what measures in medicine could be implemented to improve the health of many people. I wanted this additional educational background because

I thought it would have some value in looking at and interpreting disease data and vaccine statistics. As a practicing physician delivering babies, I felt it was important to widen my perspective on this.

By 1976, several doctors had joined my Homefirst practice. Three of them have remained with me for more than 20 years. We delivered hundreds of babies every year. We also provided healthcare. At that time, about half of the families who came to us did not vaccinate their children. (Today, it is less than one percent.) However, even the families that vaccinated chose a modified schedule. We didn't start any vaccines until six months of age, and we would never give anyone a vaccine if they were even remotely ill.

By the 1990s, the vaccine issue was becoming more prominent. I had already written thousands of medical waivers for parents opposed to vaccines. Every state has a law that the doctor can write a waiver. I would write them since I believed that vaccines were medically contraindicated. However, the law also said that the school board had a right to send parents to another doctor for a second opinion. I started getting calls from school nurses saying they were sending these children to another doctor. The second opinion was always a rubber stamp claiming there's no medical contraindication. Even *death* is not a contraindication to vaccines.

I realized this was becoming a legal issue so I enrolled in the Law School at John Marshall in Chicago. I was 49 years old at the time. John Marshall is aimed at professionals: bankers, insurance people, business owners. They have a complete night course. So, I worked full time during the day and I would go to classes at night. This went on for four years, until I received my law degree in 2000.

In law school, I wrote a paper on confidentiality. Our government doesn't have a right to probe into and control your life; that's not the role of government. So, my paper looked at who you can give confidential information to without worrying about whether it will be divulged to a third party. Clergymen have the strongest protection under the law. You can also talk freely with your lawyer. However, doctors have violated the Hippocratic Oath, which states that you will not reveal anything that a patient tells you in confidence. For example, assume a parent brings a six-month-old child to a physician for a checkup. The physician questions the parent about the child's vaccine history. The parent, believing that her communication is privileged and confidential, acknowledges that the child has not been vaccinated. Can the doctor legally and ethically use this information against the parent? No, this should not occur. Yet some doctors, upon learning that children are not vaccinated, threaten to call Social Services for "child neglect." They also share confidential health records with insurance companies.

My practice respected the choices that parents made from day one. It is based on the realization that doctors do not have the right to make decisions for families. Our obligation is to lay out the options and let families have the final word. When it comes to healthcare—whether for vaccines, yearly physicals, mammogram screenings, pap smears—families have a right to decide. We're not here to ram our beliefs down anyone's throat. That is not why we became medical doctors.

About 15 years ago I started doing complimentary seminars, open to the public. One was on homebirth and the other was on vaccines. The homebirth seminar used to attract 130 or 140 people. The vaccine seminar brought in 50 or 60 people. We would usually have 10 or 15 pregnant women in the audience; many would have their babies at home with us. However, as time went on fewer people were showing up for the homebirth seminar and more people—100, 120, 140—were showing up for the vaccine talk. In the last 10 years, we still have the same number of pregnant women coming to the seminars, but fewer women are choosing to have their babies at home. We have thousands of families come to us who don't vaccinate their children. Frequently, they ask, "How do I avoid the hepatitis B vaccine in the hospital?" My answer is always the same: "Have the baby at home."

I do a lot of seminars around the country. Every two or three years I would speak at the La Leche League (an organization that promotes breastfeeding), sometimes as their keynote speaker. They always gave me the same topic: "Asthma and the Breastfed Child." The number of breastfed children with asthma had been growing, and it really disturbed me because I couldn't figure it out. These were women who exclusively nursed their babies. Why was there such an epidemic of asthma? Then I read a study from Australia, a small study, but it was something to look at. Babies were divided into four groups: breastfed and bottlefed, with and without vaccines. Researchers looked at respiratory illnesses. The lowest amount of respiratory illness was in the breastfed and unvaccinated group. That was expected. What was unexpected was that the next lowest amount of respiratory illness was in the bottlefed and unvaccinated group. All of a sudden I realized the problem. The next time that I spoke at a La Leche League meeting, there were mothers from all around the country who had children with asthma. I asked how many of their children were vaccinated: 100 percent were vaccinated, no exceptions.

Since 1973, our medical practice, Homefirst Health Services, has cared for more than 35,000 children who were minimally vaccinated or not vaccinated at all. A few years ago, a well-known doctor visited me to do a study on autism in unvaccinated populations. This was the first time that I really looked at the figures, and I was astounded. I realized that we didn't have any cases of autism in our unvaccinated population. This wasn't something that I had preconceptions about. It was a retrospective look at what was really going on. Even when we analyzed the records from 20 years ago when we were giving some vaccines—but not starting until at least six months of age—there was no autism. We also have virtually no asthma, allergies, respiratory illness, or diabetes in our unvaccinated children, a telltale revelation when compared to national rates.

We could do even smaller samples. For example, in the last ten years we've followed nearly four thousand children who were totally under our care. None of these children were vaccinated and none of them have autism. You would expect to see 25 or 30 cases of autism in a vaccinated population of this size. (The chapter on autism summarizes a few of the notable studies on both sides of the debate.)

I tell our families that medical interventions are often unnecessary. For example, scientists looked at whether mammograms are valuable for women between 40 and 50 years of age. Eighteen of the 20 doctors who conducted a thorough review of the literature were obstetricians and radiologists who were die-hard believers in mammograms. Their conclusion was that there is no convincing evidence that it saves even one minute of life. Scientists also looked at breast cancer treatments: mastectomy, simple mastectomy, radial mastectomy. There was no benefit on outcome of survival. They looked at ultrasound: no benefit. They are very expensive baby pictures. So, my families often ask, "Well, why am I coming to you?" I say, "Good question. You're right." Most of the families in our practice are very healthy. I attribute this, for the most part, to home-births, nonvaccination, and breastfeeding. The majority of our moms nursed their babies for at least two years.

I want to say something about alternative schedules. Our medical practice never gave the whole gamut of vaccines—DPT, polio, measles, mumps and rubella—and we never started until six months of age. Today, there are a lot more vaccines (16 different vaccines for children), so more parents now wonder whether it's better to deviate from the CDC's recommended immunization schedule. For example, some parents don't want to give the MMR shot to their children. They'd rather have the measles, mumps and rubella shots administered separately, the way they were given in the 1970s. Other parents like to choose vaccines that have the least amount of aluminum (read the chapter on aluminum). These measures are probably more sensible than taking all of the shots at once (read the chapter on multiple vaccines) or loading up the infant's developing neurological and immunological systems with high amounts of toxic additives (read the chapter on vaccine ingredients). However, you're merely mitigating the potential damage. I don't believe you're going to eliminate it altogether.

The current schedule of recommended vaccines is so crowded that doctors give babies several shots during a single office visit—up to eight or nine vaccines *all at one time.* (Babies get 38 doses by the time they are 1½ years old—see chart on the following page.) Parents, and doctors, often forget that vaccines are drugs. How often do we, as adults, take that many drugs at the same time? Would we be more surprised if we *did* or *did not* have an adverse reaction?

Parents sometimes ask, "What if my kid gets one of these diseases and I didn't have him vaccinated?" Well, the child could become ill, develop complications, or die. However, each disease is unique and has to be looked at separately. This is why every chapter in this book describes the prevalence of each disease and who is most at risk. Let me tell you something, though: a whole lot of people are injured and killed from vaccines. You will learn about these possibilities as well. There are no guarantees.

Authorities claim that vaccines reduced the incidence of disease. However, several diseases—tuberculosis, scarlet fever, plague—infected thousands of people every year but virtually disappeared without any vaccines. How do we explain this? Doctors also claim that parents have a duty to vaccinate their children to protect all of the other kids in the community (read the chapter on Social Obligation). They call this herd immunity. However, this assumes that vaccines work as intended. In this book you will learn how efficacy is measured. In the past few years we have seen outbreaks of measles, mumps and pertussis in mostly vaccinated children. Studies show that immunity from the chickenpox vaccine doesn't last very long, and recently vaccinated children can spread the disease to other people. Authorities call these "secondary transmissions." In Africa, the oral polio vaccine is *causing* polio. This was a problem in the United States until they stopped administering this live-virus vaccine.

The FDA and CDC allow important vaccine studies to be conducted by the pharmaceutical companies that make and sell the vaccines being studied. This is like asking foxes to guard the henhouse. You'll rarely read something written by a pediatrician admitting to the true side effects of vaccines. These are documented in numerous studies. Instead, most doctors will recommend that your child receive every available vaccine, under nearly every condition, with few exceptions.

Do Babies Get Too Many Vaccines?

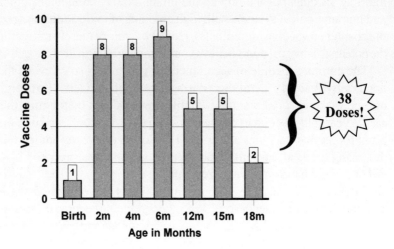

Today, children receive one vaccine at birth, eight vaccines at two months, eight vaccines at four months, nine vaccines at six months, and twelve additional vaccines between 12 and18 months—38 drug doses by the time they are 1½ years old! Source: CDC, *Recommended Immunization Schedule 2010.*

A free society believes in freedom of speech and the right to learn as much about vaccines as possible. There should be no restriction on the information that you have access to, and everyone should be free to accept or reject vaccines. I don't recommend for or against the shots. The information that I am presenting here is to help you look at the scientific literature. Hundreds of important vaccine studies are summarized in this book. Many of them are critical of vaccines. Therefore, this book should be considered supplemental to other information that you gather from both "official" and alternative sources.

As parents, all of us are concerned about our children and grandchildren. We want to do what's absolutely in their best interest. However, the right course of action is not always clear. Is the industry mantra—that vaccine benefits outweigh risks—an established fact or merely an effective marketing tool? After reading this book, I believe you will be more qualified to *Make an Informed Vaccine Decision for the Health of Your Child.*

Mayer Eisenstein, MD, JD, MPH
Medical Director, Homefirst® Health Services

Polio

What is polio?

Polio is a contagious disease caused by an intestinal virus that may attack nerve cells of the brain and spinal cord. Symptoms include fever, headache, sore throat, and vomiting. Some victims develop neurological complications, including stiffness of the neck and back, weak muscles, pain in the joints, and paralysis of one or more limbs or respiratory muscles. In severe cases it may be fatal, due to respiratory paralysis.

How is polio contracted?

Polio can be spread through contact with contaminated feces (for example, by changing an infected baby's diapers) or through airborne droplets, in food, or in water. The virus enters the body by nose or mouth, then travels to the intestines where it incubates. Next, it enters the bloodstream where "anti-polio" antibodies are produced. In most cases, this stops progression of the virus and the individual gains permanent immunity against the disease.

How prevalent and serious is polio?

Many people mistakenly believe that anyone who contracts polio will become paralyzed or die. However, in most infections caused by polio there are few distinctive symptoms.[1] In fact, 95 percent of everyone who is exposed to the natural polio virus won't exhibit any symptoms, even under epidemic conditions.[2] About five percent of infected people will experience mild symptoms, such as a sore throat, stiff neck, headache, and fever—often diagnosed as a cold or flu. Muscular paralysis has been estimated to occur in about one of every 1,000 people who contract the disease.[3] This has lead some scientific researchers to conclude that the small percentage of people who do develop paralytic polio may be anatomically susceptible to the disease. The vast remainder of the population may be naturally immune to the polio virus.

Paralytic polio is rarely permanent. Usually there is a full recovery. Muscle power begins to return after several days and continues to improve during the next 12-24 months. A small percentage of cases will experience residual paralysis. In rare cases, paralysis of the muscles used to breathe can lead to death.[4-8]

The DPT Vaccine and Other Shots
Could Cause Polio

When diphtheria and pertussis vaccines were introduced in the 1940s, cases of paralytic polio skyrocketed. This was documented in *The Lancet* and other medical journals.[9-12] In 1949, the Medical Research Council in Great Britain set up a committee to investigate the matter and ultimately concluded that people are at increased risk of paralysis for 30 days following injections.[13,14]

A 1992 study, published in the *Journal of Infectious Diseases,* validated earlier findings. Children who received DPT (diphtheria, tetanus, and pertussis) injections were significantly more likely than controls to suffer paralytic poliomyelitis within the next 30 days. According to the authors, "this study confirms that injections are an important cause of provocative poliomyelitis."[15]

In 1995, the *New England Journal of Medicine* published a study showing that children who received a single injection within one month after receiving a polio vaccine were eight times more likely to contract polio than children who received no injections.[16] These studies and others indicate that "injections must be avoided in countries with endemic poliomyelitis."[17]

Can polio be treated?
Treatment mainly consists of putting the patient to bed and allowing the affected limbs to be completely relaxed. If breathing is affected, a respirator or iron lung can be used. Physical therapy may be required.

The polio vaccine:
In 1952, Jonas Salk, an American microbiologist, combined three types of polio virus grown in cultures made from monkey kidneys. Using formaldehyde, he was able to "kill" or inactivate the viral matter so that it would trigger an antibody response without causing the disease. That year he began his initial experiments on human subjects. In 1953, his findings were printed in the *Journal of the American Medical Association.*[18] In April 1955, the nation's first polio immunization campaign was launched. Shortly thereafter, 70,000 school children became seriously ill from Salk's vaccine—the infamous "Cutter Incident." Many of these children contracted polio from the vaccine, were paralyzed and died. Apparently, Salk's "killed-virus" vaccine was not fully inactivated.[19,20] The vaccine was redeveloped, and by August 1955 over 4 million doses were administered in the United States. By 1959, nearly 100 other countries were using Salk's vaccine.

Nutritional Deficiencies Could Increase the Risk of Polio

A poor diet has been shown to raise susceptibility to polio.[21] In 1948, during the height of the polio epidemics, Dr. Benjamin Sandler, a nutritional expert at the Oteen Veterans' Hospital, documented a link between polio and an excessive use of sugars and starches. He compiled records showing that countries with the highest per capita consumption of sugar, such as the United States, Britain, Australia, Canada, and Sweden (with over 100 pounds per person per year) had the greatest incidence of polio. In contrast, polio was practically unheard of in China (with its sugar use of only 3 pounds per person per year).[22]

Dr. Sandler claimed that sugars and starches lower blood sugar levels causing hypoglycemia, and that phosphoric acid in soft drinks strips the nerves of proper nourishment. Such foods dehydrate the cells and leech calcium from the body. A serious calcium deficiency precedes polio. Weakened nerve trunks are then more likely to malfunction and the victim loses the use of one or more limbs.[23-25]

In 1957, Albert Sabin, another American scientist, developed a live-virus (oral) vaccine against polio. He didn't think Salk's killed-virus vaccine would be effective at preventing epidemics. He wanted his vaccine to simulate a real-life infection. This meant using an attenuated or weakened form of the live virus. He experimented with thousands of monkeys and chimpanzees before isolating a rare type of polio virus that would reproduce in the intestinal tract without penetrating the central nervous system. The initial human trials were conducted in foreign countries. In 1958, it was tested in the United States. In 1963, Sabin's oral "sugar-cube" vaccine became available for general use.

Which vaccine is in use today?

In 1963, Sabin's oral vaccine quickly replaced Salk's injectable shot. It is cheaper to make, easier to take, and appears to provide greater protection, including "herd immunity" in unvaccinated people. However, it cannot be given to people with weak immune systems. Plus, it is capable of causing polio in some recipients of the vaccine, and in people with weak immune systems who come into close contact with recently vaccinated children.[26] Thus, in 2000 the CDC "updated" its U.S. polio vaccine recommendations reverting back to policies first implemented during the 1950s. The oral vaccine should only be used in "special circumstances."

(Several countries still use the live-virus, oral vaccine.) Otherwise, children should be given the inactivated polio vaccine (IPV):

- Ipol (the inactivated or killed-virus shot)—A "sterile suspension of three types of poliovirus...grown in Vero cells, a continuous line of monkey kidney cells cultivated on microcarriers." The cells are "supplemented with newborn calf serum." Each dose also contains 2-phenoxyethanol, formaldehyde, neomycin, streptomycin and polymyxin B. Produced by Sanofi Pasteur. Given in four doses.[27]

Other combination vaccines with IPV are available, including: Kinrix (DTaP/Polio); Pediarix (DTaP/Polio/Hep B); and Pentacel (DTaP/Polio/Hib).

Safety

In 1976, Dr. Jonas Salk, creator of the killed-virus vaccine used in the 1950s, testified that the live-virus vaccine (used almost exclusively in the U.S. from the early 1960s to 2000) was the "principal if not sole cause" of all reported polio cases in the U.S. since 1961.[28] In 1992, the CDC acknowledged that the live-virus vaccine had become the dominant cause of polio in the U.S.[29] Public outrage at these tragedies became the impetus for removing the oral polio vaccine from immunization schedules.

The following story is a firsthand account of one man's experience after his son received the oral polio vaccine:

"Four months ago my son was taken to a local clinic for his polio vaccine. Unfortunately, he changed from that day—high-pitched screaming, smelly stools, non-stop crying, difficulty in breathing, high temperature, and lethargy. He also lost weight. Weeks of sleepless nights for all of us followed. His development ceased. He had been able to stand and move around, but he went back to remaining in basically whatever position we left him in. My wife was six months pregnant at the time, and about a week after our son's polio vaccine, she began to have headaches, loss of balance, muscular weakness, and frequent tiredness. I panicked because everything seemed to be pointing to polio infection. Then, a week after her continuous headaches began, she had to go to the hospital because there was something wrong with the pregnancy; she lost our daughter. I tried to get a polio test, and to find the cause of this tragic series of events, but the medical profession was extremely unhelpful. They laughed at me. I will never know why our son suddenly stopped growing or why his development regressed. I will never know why we lost our daughter. The thing I am sure about is that the precursor to these events was the polio vaccine."[30]

How safe is the current inactivated polio vaccine?

A fact sheet on polio published by the U.S. Department of Health and Human Services warns parents that the inactivated polio vaccine (IPV) can cause "serious problems *or even death*."[31] Product information published by the IPV manufacturer notes that "although no causal relationship has been established, deaths have occurred in temporal association after vaccination of infants with IPV."[32] The IPV manufacturer also warns that Guillain-Barré syndrome (a debilitating ailment characterized by muscular incapacitation, paralysis, and nervous system damage—symptoms that are virtually indistinguishable from polio) "has been temporally related to administration of another inactivated poliovirus vaccine."[33] Yet, despite these danger alerts, medical authorities continue to assure parents that the currently available inactivated polio vaccine is both safe and effective.

The case reports on the next page were taken directly from the FDA's Vaccine Adverse Event Reporting System (VAERS).[34] They are just a small sample of the potential side effects associated with the inactivated, or killed-virus, polio vaccine. (Case numbers precede report summaries.)

Efficacy

Polio is virtually nonexistent in the United States today. However, according to Dr. Robert Mendelsohn, there is no credible scientific evidence that the vaccine caused polio to disappear.[35] From 1923 to 1953, *before* the polio vaccine was introduced, the polio death rate in the United States and England had already declined on its own by 47 percent and 55 percent, respectively.[36] Statistics show a similar decline in other European countries as well. In addition, when the vaccine did become available, many European countries questioned its effectiveness and refused to systematically inoculate their citizens. Yet, polio epidemics also ended in these countries.[37]

The standards for defining polio were changed when the polio vaccine was introduced. The new definition of a polio epidemic required more cases to be reported. Paralytic polio was redefined as well, making it more difficult to confirm and tally cases. Prior to the introduction of the vaccine the patient only had to exhibit paralytic symptoms for 24 hours. Laboratory confirmation and tests to determine residual paralysis were not required. The new definition required the patient to exhibit paralytic symptoms for at least 60 days, and residual paralysis had to be confirmed twice during the course of the disease. Also, after the vaccine was introduced cases of aseptic meningitis (an infectious disease difficult to distinguish from polio) and coxsackie virus infections were more often reported as separate

---

Inactivated Polio Vaccine (IPV)—VAERS Case Reports

▸112738: A 4-month-old girl received IPV, fell asleep, and upon awakening "had a sick sounding cry and did not have control of facial muscles." Her face was drooping and she could not smile.

▸160203: A 4-month-old girl received IPV, had cardiac arrest and died the following day.

▸209102: A one-year-old boy received his 3rd dose of inactivated polio vaccine and later that day started having seizures. He was rushed to the hospital and intubated. The child was transferred to the pediatric intensive care unit for additional treatment.

▸234886: A 5-year-old girl received the inactivated polio vaccine and one week later developed polydipsia and polyuria (excessive thirst and urination). She was subsequently diagnosed with insulin dependent diabetes mellitus (IDDM), hyperglycemia, and immune disorder.

---

diseases from polio. But such cases were counted as polio before the vaccine was introduced. The vaccine's reported effectiveness was therefore skewed.[38]

Dr. Bernard Greenberg, chairman of the Committee on Evaluation and Standards of the American Public Health Association during the 1950s, confirmed that dubious tactics were used to fabricate polio vaccine efficacy rates. His expert testimony was used as evidence during congressional hearings in 1962. He credited the "decline" of polio cases not to the vaccine, but rather to a change in the way doctors were required to report cases:

"Prior to 1954, any physician who reported paralytic poliomyelitis was doing his patient a service by way of subsidizing the cost of hospitalization. In 1955, the criteria were changed. This meant that we started reporting a new disease. Furthermore, diagnostic procedures have continued to be refined. Coxsackie virus infections and aseptic meningitis have been distinguished from poliomyelitis. Thus, simply by changes in diagnostic criteria, the number of paralytic cases was predetermined to decrease."[39]

—Bernard Greenberg, MD, testifying before Congress

How effective is the current polio vaccine?

In studies designed to measure efficacy of the current inactivated polio vaccine, "serum neutralizing antibodies" were detected in 84 percent to 100 percent of infants after receiving two doses of the vaccine. Rates were higher after the third and fourth doses. According to the manufacturer, a "survey" of Swedish children who received IPV in the 1970s demonstrated "persistence of neutralizing antibody" for at least ten years.[40]

Impure Polio Vaccines

Several different animal viruses contaminated early polio vaccines, which were administered to millions of people throughout the world. Studies and other evidence appear to confirm that increasing rates of previously rare diseases may be related to these tainted shots. This has led some researchers to wonder whether we are trading polio for cancer and other immunological disorders.

Polio vaccines and CANCER:

In 1959, Bernice Eddy, a brilliant government scientist working in Biologics at the National Institutes of Health, discovered that polio vaccines being administered throughout the world contained an infectious agent capable of causing cancer. When Eddy attempted to report her findings and halt production of these contaminated polio vaccines, her government superiors barred her from publicly revealing the problem. Instead, her lab and equipment were taken away and she was demoted.[41,42]

In 1960, Drs. Ben Sweet and M.R. Hilleman, pharmaceutical researchers for the Merck Institute for Therapeutic Research, were credited with discovering this infectious agent—SV-40, a monkey virus that infected nearly all rhesus monkeys, whose kidneys were used to produce polio vaccines. Hilleman and Sweet found SV-40 in all three types of Albert Sabin's live oral polio vaccine, and noted the possibility that it might cause cancer, "especially when administered to human babies."[43,44] According to Sweet, "It was a frightening discovery because, back then, it was not possible to detect the virus with the testing procedures we had.... We had no idea of what this virus would do." Sweet elaborated:

"First, we knew that SV-40 had oncogenic properties in hamsters, which was bad news. Secondly, we found out that it hybridized with certain DNA viruses...such that [they] would then have SV-40 genes attached [to them].... When we started growing the vaccines, we just couldn't get rid of the SV-40-contaminated virus. We tried to neutralize it, but couldn't.... Now, with the theoretical links to HIV and cancer, it just blows my mind."[45]
—Ben Sweet, MD, co-finder of SV-40 in the polio vaccine

Further research into SV-40 uncovered even more disturbing information. This cancer-causing virus was not only ingested via Sabin's contaminated oral sugar-cube vaccine, but was directly injected into people's bloodstreams as well. Apparently, SV-40 survived the formaldehyde Salk used to kill microbes that defiled his injectable vaccine.[46,47] Experts estimate that between 1954 and 1963, 30 million to 100 million Americans and perhaps another 100 million or more people throughout the world were exposed to SV-40 through ill-conceived polio eradication campaigns.[48]

Numerous studies published in eminent journals throughout the world appear to confirm that SV-40 is a catalyst for many types of cancer.[49-68] It has been found in brain tumors and leukemia.[69] Michele Carbone, a molecular pathologist at Chicago's Loyola University Medical Center, was able to detect SV-40 in 38 percent of patients with bone cancer and in 58 percent of those with mesothelioma, a deadly type of lung cancer.[70-72] Carbone's research indicates that SV-40 blocks an important protein that normally protects cells from becoming malignant.[73]

In 1998, a national cancer database was analyzed: 17 percent more bone cancers, 20 percent more brain cancers, and 178 percent more mesotheliomas were found in people who were exposed to SV-40-tainted polio vaccines.[74] The National Institutes of Health created a map showing the geographic distribution of contaminated stock.[75] Using this map, researchers found osteosarcoma bone tumor rates to be 10 times higher than normal in some regions where this tainted vaccine was used.[76,77]

Perhaps the most alarming aspect of this ongoing simian virus debacle can be found in other studies suggesting that SV-40, introduced to humans through the polio vaccine, can be passed from human to human and from mother to child. A study of nearly 59,000 women found that children of mothers who received the Salk vaccine between 1959 and 1965 had brain tumors at a rate 13 times greater than mothers who did not receive those polio shots.[78-80]

Another study published in the medical journal *Cancer Research* found SV-40 present in 23 percent of blood samples and 45 percent of semen taken from healthy subjects.[81,82] Apparently, the virus is being spread sexually and from mother to child in the womb. According to biology and genetics professor Mauro Tognon, one of the study's authors, this would explain why brain, bone, and lung cancers are on the rise—a 30 percent increase in U.S. brain tumors alone during a recent 25-year period—and why SV-40 was detected in brain tumors of children born after 1965 who did not receive polio vaccines containing the virus.[83]

Despite official denials of any correlation between SV-40-contaminated polio vaccines and increased cancer rates, more than 62 papers from 30 laboratories around the world have reported SV-40 in human tissues and tumors. The virus was also discovered in pituitary and thyroid tumors, and in patients with kidney disease.[84] Even the National Cancer Institute issued a statement that SV-40 "may be associated with human cancer."[85]

Polio vaccines and AIDS:

SV-40, the cancer-causing monkey virus found in polio vaccines and administered to millions of unsuspecting people throughout the world, was just one of numerous simian viruses known to have contaminated polio vaccines. For example, Dr. Hilary Koprowski, an early vaccine researcher, wrote the following to a congressional panel studying the safety of growing live polio-virus vaccine in monkey kidneys:

> *"As monkey kidney culture is host to innumerable simian viruses, the number found varying in relation to the amount of work expended to find them, the problem presented to the manufacturer is considerable, if not insuperable. As our technical methods improve we may find fewer and fewer lots of vaccine which can be called free from simian virus."*[86]
> **—Hilary Koprowski, MD**

According to Harvard Medical School professor Ronald Desrosier, the practice of growing polio vaccines in monkey kidneys is "a ticking time bomb."[87] Evidently, some viruses can live inside monkeys without causing harm. But if these viruses were to somehow cross species and enter the human population, new diseases could occur. Desrosier continued:

> *"The danger in using monkey tissue to produce human vaccines is that some viruses produced by monkeys may be transferred to humans in the vaccine, with very bad health consequences."*[88]
> **—Ronald Desrosier, MD, Harvard professor**

Desrosier also warns that testing can only be done for known viruses, and that our knowledge is limited to about "2 percent of existing monkey viruses."[89] Craig Engesser of Lederle Laboratories acknowledged that "you can't test for something if you don't know it's there."[90] Virus detection techniques were crude and unreliable during the 1950s, 60s, and 70s when polio vaccines were initially produced. It wasn't until the mid 1980s that new and more sophisticated testing procedures were developed.[91] That was when researchers discovered that about half of all African green monkeys—the preferred primate for making polio vaccines—were infected with simian immunodeficiency virus (SIV), a virus closely related to human immunodeficiency virus (HIV), the infectious agent thought to precede AIDS.[92-95] This caused some researchers to wonder whether HIVs may simply be SIVs "residing in and adapting to a human host."[96] Others suspected that SIV may have mutated into HIV once it was introduced into the human population by way of contaminated polio vaccines.[97-101]

Vaccine authorities were so concerned about the possibility that SIV was a precursor to HIV, and that polio vaccines were the means of transmission from monkey to human, that the World Health Organization (WHO) convened two meetings of experts in 1985 to explore the data and consider their options.[102-104] After all, SIV was very similar to HIV and occurred naturally in the monkey species predominantly used by vaccine manufacturers.[105] Nevertheless, WHO concluded that the vaccines were safe and insisted that vaccination campaigns should continue unabated.

Japanese researchers conducted their own investigation and found that African green monkeys used to produce polio vaccines had antibodies against SIV. The implication was clear: monkeys used to produce polio vaccines were natural carriers of a virus that looked and acted like HIV, the infectious agent linked to AIDS. In 1989, they recommended that monkeys infected with SIV not be used to make polio vaccines.[106]

In 1990, wild chimpanzees in Africa were found to be infected with a strain of SIV that was nearly identical to HIV.[107] Some researchers called it "the missing link" to the origins of human immunodeficiency virus.[108] And since chimpanzees were used to test viruses for potential use in vaccines, and were kept in captivity by research laboratories, they could have been a source of vaccine contamination.[109,110] Scientific concerns were also heightened when researchers found some West Africans who were infected with an SIV-like virus that was a fundamental twin to HIV. They called it HIV-2, and like the initial HIV subtype, it was implicated in the development of AIDS.[111] According to Robert Gallo, an expert on the AIDS virus, some versions of the SIV monkey virus are virtually indistinguishable from some human variants of HIV:

> *"The monkey virus is the human virus. There are monkey viruses as close to isolates of HIV-2 as HIV-2 isolates are to each other."*[112]
> **—Robert Gallo, MD, AIDS expert**

More animal viruses:

Thousands of viruses and other potentially infectious microorganisms thrive in monkeys and cows, the preferred animals for making polio vaccines.[113] SV-40, SIV, and BSE (bovine spongiform encephalopathy, or Mad Cow disease) are just three of the disease-causing agents researchers have investigated. For example, scientists have known since 1955 that monkeys host the "B" virus, foamy agent virus, haemadsorption viruses, the LCM virus, arboviruses, and more.[114] Bovine immunodeficiency virus (BIV), similar in gene structure to HIV, was recently found in some cows.[115]

In 1956, respiratory syncytial virus (RSV) was found in chimpanzees.[116] According to Dr. Viera Scheibner, vaccine researcher, RSV viruses "formed prominent contaminants in polio vaccines, and were soon detected in children."[117] They caused serious cold-like symptoms in small infants and babies who received the polio vaccine.

Dr. John Martin, a professor of pathology at the University of Southern California, has been warning authorities since 1978 that other dangerous monkey viruses could be contaminating polio vaccines. In particular, Martin sought to investigate simian cytomegalovirus (SCMV), a "stealth virus" capable of causing neurological disorders in the human brain. The virus was found in monkeys used for making polio vaccines. The government rebuffed his efforts to study the risks. However, in 1995 Martin published his findings implicating the African green monkey as the probable source of SCMV isolated from a patient with chronic fatigue syndrome.[118]

In 1996, Dr. Howard B. Urnovitz, a microbiologist, founder and chief science officer of Calypte Biomedical in Berkeley, California spoke at a national AIDS conference where he revealed that up to 26 monkey viruses may have been in the original Salk vaccines. These included the simian equivalents of human echo virus, coxsackie, herpes (HHV-6, HHV-7, and HHV-8), adenoviruses, Epstein-Barr, and cytomegalovirus.[119-121] Urnovitz believes that contaminated Salk vaccines given to U.S. children between 1955 and 1961 may have set this generation up for immune system damage and neurological disorders. He sees correlations between early polio vaccine campaigns and the sudden emergence of human T-cell leukemia, epidemic Kaposi's sarcoma, Burkitt's lymphoma, herpes, Epstein-Barr and chronic fatigue syndrome.[122]

Worldwide polio eradication:

By 2007, worldwide polio eradication remained an elusive goal. Cases were recorded in at least 16 countries, most notably in Nigeria, India, Pakistan, Somalia and Afghanistan.[123] It should also be noted that some children in foreign regions of the world are receiving "more than 12 doses of [polio] vaccine before their second birthday," yet they are still susceptible to the disease. For example, in India "a median of 10 reported vaccine doses have been received by persons who have contracted poliomyelitis; this has raised questions about the efficacy of the vaccine."[124] Poor nutrition has been proposed as one possible reason many children are not developing immunity to polio after receiving multiple doses of the vaccine. At any rate, a precise timeline for polio eradication "remains unpredictable."[125]

Animal tissue vs. human cells:

Despite the polio vaccine's long history of causing polio, and the FDA's inability to protect the public from dangerous contaminants, the currently available inactivated or "killed-virus" polio vaccine continues to be manufactured in much the same way as earlier versions; monkey kidneys, calf serum, and toxic chemicals are still used.[126] In Canada, the inactivated polio vaccine is made in "human diploid cells" instead of monkey kidneys. According to Barbara Loe Fisher, president of the National Vaccine Information Center: "With mounting evidence that cross-species transfer of viruses can occur, the U.S. should no longer be using animal tissues to produce vaccines."[127] However, Dr. Arthur Levine of the National Institutes of Health believes that making polio vaccines with human cells isn't risk-free either, "because they must be tested for human infections."[128]

Are positive changes possible?

Government officials worry that even debating the issue will frighten parents. Levine probably speaks for many people within the vaccine industry when he declares: "We do a grave disservice to the public if we were now to question the safety of the current polio vaccines...."[129] But Barbara Loe Fisher would like to see changes in the way vaccine safety is governed. She believes that agencies like the FDA have an inherent conflict of interest because of their mandate to promote universal vaccination on the one hand and regulate vaccine safety on the other:

> *"Who's minding the store when the FDA has allowed drug companies to produce vaccines grown on contaminated monkey kidneys? What happened to protecting the public health?"*[130]
> —**Barbara Loe Fisher, vaccine safety advocate**

Dr. John Martin agrees. He believes that we need to immediately determine the prevalence of stealth viruses of simian origin in the United States, and whether they may be contributing to chronic immune system and brain disorders in children and adults.[131] Dr. Urnovitz is even more resolute in his convictions. He thinks that an extensive study of human exposure to simian microbes is long overdue:

> *"Half of the people in this country are baby boomers born between 1941 and 1961 and are at high risk for having been exposed to polio vaccines contaminated with monkey viruses. Are we just a time bomb waiting to happen, waiting to develop lupus, Alzheimer's and Parkinson's disease?"*[132]
> —**Howard B. Urnovitz, MD, microbiologist**

Urnovitz also challenged medical science to prove him wrong: "What we are saying here is that there is a strong probability that no human retroviruses existed before the polio vaccines. You have to realize that if you mess around with nature, you're going to pay the price. The objective here is a better, healthier world."[133]

Notes

1. Volk, WA., et al. *Basic Microbiology, 4th edition.* (Philadelphia, PA: J.B. Lippincott Co., 1980):455.

2. Burnet, M., et al. *The Natural History of Infectious Disease* (New York, NY: Cambridge University Press, 1972):16.

3. Sanofi Pasteur. "IPOL® (Poliovirus Vaccine Inactivated)." Product insert from the vaccine manufacturer. December 2005.

4. Harry, NM. "The recovery period in anterior poliomyelitis." *British Medical Journal* 1938;1:164–7.

5. Sharrard, W. "Muscle recovery in poliomyelitis." *J Bone Joint Surgery* 1955; 37B:63–79.

6. Affeldt, JE., et al. "Functional and vocational recovery in severe poliomyelitis." *Clinical Orthopaedics and Related Research* 1958;12:16–21.

7. Hollenberg, C., et al. "The late effects of spinal poliomyelitis." *Canadian Medical Association Journal* 1959;81:343–6.

8. Ramlow, J., et al. "Epidemiology of the post-polio syndrome." *American Journal of Epidemiology* 1992;136:783.

9. Lindsay, KW., et al. *Neurology and Neurosurgery Illustrated.* (Edinburgh/London/New York: Churchill Livingston, 1986):100, Figure 15.2. Polio incidence rates obtained from National Morbidity Reports.

10. McCloskey, BP. "The relation of prophylactic inoculations to the onset of poliomyelitis." *The Lancet* (April 18, 1950):659–63.

11. Geffen, DH. "The incidence of paralysis occurring in London children within four weeks after immunization." *Med Officer* 1950;83:137–40.

12. Martin, JK. "Local paralysis in children after injections." *Arch Dis Child* 1950;25:1–14.

13. Hill, AB., et al. "Inoculation and poliomyelitis. A statistical investigation in England and Wales in 1949." *British Medical Journal* 1950;ii:1–6.

14. Medical Research Council Committee on Inoculation Procedures and Neurological Lesions. "Poliomyelitis and prophylactic inoculation." *The Lancet* 1956;ii:1223–31.

15. Sutter, RW., et al. "Attributable risk of DTP (diphtheria and tetanus toxoids and pertussis vaccine) injection in provoking paralytic poliomyelitis during a large outbreak in Oman." *J of Infectious Diseases* 1992; 165:444–9.

16. Strebel, PM., et al. "Intramuscular injections within 30 days of immunization with oral poliovirus vaccine—a risk factor for vaccine-associated paralytic poliomyelitis." *New England J of Med* (February 23, 1995):500+.

17. Editorial. "Provocation paralysis." *Lancet* 1992;340:1005.

18. Salk, J., et al. "Studies in human subjects on active immunization against poliomyelitis. A preliminary report of experiments in progress." *JAMA* 1953; 151(13):1081-98.

19. Offit, P. *The Cutter Incident* (Yale University Press, 2005).

20. Offit, P. "The Cutter Incident: 50 Years Later." *New England Journal of Medicine* 2005;352:1411-1412.

21. Chandra, RK. "Reduced secretory antibody response to live attenuated measles and poliovirus vaccines in malnourished children." *British Medical Journal* 1975;ii:583–5.

22. McBean, E. *The Poisoned Needle* (Mokelumne Hill, California: Health Research, 1957):116-118;146.

23. Sandler, B. *American J of Pathology* (January 1941).

24. Sandler, B. *Diet Prevents Polio* (Milwaukee: Lee Foundation for Nutrition Research, 1951).

25. Allen, H. *Don't Get Stuck: The Case Against Vaccinations* (Oldsmar, Florida: Natural Hygiene Press, 1985):166.

26. Strebel, PM., et al. "Epidemiology of poliomyelitis in U.S. one decade after the last reported case of indigenous wild virus associated disease." *Clinical Infectious Diseases,* CDC (February 1992):568–79.

27. See Note 3.

28. *Washington Post* (September 24, 1976).

29. See Note 26.

30. Thinktwice Global Vaccine Institute. Unsolicited case report submitted by a concerned parent. www.thinktwice.com

31. CDC. "Polio: what you need to know." *U.S. Department of Health and Human Services* (October 15, 1991):3.

32. See Note 3.

33. Ibid.

34. National Vaccine Information Center. "MedAlerts: access to the U.S. government's Vaccine Adverse Event Reporting System (VAERS)." www.medalerts.org

35. Mendelsohn, R. *How to Raise a Healthy Child...In Spite of Your Doctor* (Ballantine Books, 1984):231.

36. Alderson, M. *International Mortality Statistics* (Wash., DC: Facts on File, 1981):177–8.

37. See Note 35.

38. Hearings Before the Committee on Interstate and Foreign Commerce, House of Representatives, 87th Congress, 2nd Session on HR 10541 (May 1962):94–112.

39. Ibid., pp. 96-97.

40. See Note 3.

41. O'Hern, M. *Profiles: Pioneer Women Scientists.* Bethesda, MD: National Institutes of Health.

42. Curtis, T., et al. "Scientist's polio fear unheeded: how U.S. researcher's warning was silenced." *The Houston Post* 1992:A1 and A12.

43. Ibid.

44. Sweet, BH., Hilleman MR. "The vacuolating virus: SV-40." As cited in: "The polio vaccine and simian virus 40," by Moriarty, TJ. www.vaccinationnews.com/DailyNews/June2001/PolioVaxSV40.htm

45. Moriarty TJ. "The polio vaccine and simian virus 40." *Vaccination News.* www.vaccinationnews.com/DailyNews/June2001/PolioVaxSV40.htm

46. Shah, K., et al. "Human exposure to SV40." *American J Epidem* 1976;103:1-12.

47. Curtis, T. "The origin of AIDS: A startling new theory attempts to answer the question 'Was it an act of God or an act of man?'" *Rolling Stone* (March 19, 1992):57.

48. Bookchin, D., et al. "Tainted polio vaccine still carries its threat 40 years later." *The Boston Globe* (January 26, 1997). Also see Notes 46 and 47.

49. Innis, MD. "Oncogenesis and poliomyelitis vaccine." *Nature* 1968;219:972–3.

50. Soriano, F., et al. "Simian virus 40 in a human cancer." *Nature* 1974;249: 421–4.

51. Weiss, AF., et al. "Simian virus 40-related antigens in three human meningiomas with defined chromosome loss." *Proceedings of the Nat Academy of Science* 1975; 72(2):609–13.

52. Scherneck, S., et al. "Isolation of a SV-40-like papovavirus from a human glioblastoma." *International Journal of Cancer* 1979;24:523–31.

53. Stoian, M., et al. "Possible relation between viruses and oromaxillofacial tumors.

II. Research on the presence of SV-40 antigen and specific antibodies in patients with oromaxillofacial tumors." *Virologie* 1987;38:35–40.

54. Stoian, M., et al. "Possible relation between viruses and oromaxillofacial tumors. II. Detection of SV40 antigen and of anti-SV40 antibodies in patients with parotid gland tumors." *Virologie* 1987;38:41–6.

55. Bravo, MP., et al. "Association between the occurrence of antibodies to simian vacuolating virus 40 and bladder cancer in male smokers. *Neoplasma* 1988;35:285–8.

56. O'Connell, K., et al. "Endothelial cells transformed by SV40 T-antigen cause Kaposi's sarcoma-like tumors in nude mice." *American Journal of Pathology* 1991;139(4):743–9.

57. Weiner, LP., et al. "Isolation of virus related to SV40 from patients with progressive multifocal leukoencephalopathy." *New England Journal of Medicine* 1972;286:385–90.

58. Tabuchi, K. "Screening of human brain tumors for SV-40-related T-antigen." *International Journal of Cancer* 1978;21:12–7.

59. Meinke, W., et al. "Simian virus 40-related DNA sequences in a human brain tumor." *Neurology* 1979;29:1590–4.

60. Krieg, P., et al. "Episomal simian virus 40 genomes in human brain tumors." *Proceedings of the National Academy of Science* 1981;78:6446-50.

61. Krieg, P., et al. "Cloning of SV40 genomes from human brain tumors." *Virology* 1984;138:336–40.

62. Geissler, E. "SV40 in human intracranial tumors: passenger virus or oncogenic 'hit-and-run' agent?" *Z Klin Med* 1986;41:493–5.

63. Geissler, E. "SV40 and human brain tumors." *Prog in Med Virology* 1990;37: 211–22.

64. Bergsagel, DJ., et al. "DNA sequences similar to those of simian virus 40 in ependymomas and choroid plexus tumors of childhood." *New England J of Medicine* 1992;326:988–93.

65. Martini, M., et al. "Human brain tumors and simian virus 40." *Journal of the National Cancer Institute* 1995;87(17):1331.

66. Lednicky, JA., et al. "Natural simian virus 40 strains are present in human choroid plexus and ependymoma tumors." *Virology* 1995;212(2):710–7.

67. Tognon, M., et al. "Large T antigen coding sequence of two DNA tumor viruses, BK and SV-40, and nonrandom chromosome changes in two gioblastoma cell lines." *Cancer Genetics and Cytogenics* 1996;90(1): 17–23.

68. Vilchez, RA., et al. "Association between simian virus 40 and non-hodgkin lymphoma." *The Lancet* (March 9, 2002);359: 817–23.

69. See Notes 57-68.

70. Carbone, M., et al. "SV-40-like sequences in human bone tumors." *Oncogene* 1996; 13(3):527–35.

71. Pass, HI., Carbone, M., et al. "Evidence for and implications of SV-40-like sequences in human mesotheliomas." *Important Advances in Oncology* 1996:89-108.

72. Rock, A. "The lethal dangers of the billion dollar vaccine business." *Money* (December 1996):161.

73. Ibid.

74. Carlsen, W. "Rogue virus in the vaccine: Early polio vaccine harbored virus now feared to cause cancer in humans." *San Francisco Chronicle* (July 15, 2001):7. Research by Susan Fisher, epidemiologist, Loyola University Medical Center.

75. National Institutes of Health. Zones of contamination: Globe staff graphic.

76. Bookchin, D., et al. "Tainted polio vaccine still carries its threat 40 years later." *The Boston Globe* (January 26, 1997).

77. "SV-40 contamination of polio vaccine." *Well Within Online* (February 3, 2001). www.nccn.net/~wwithin/polio.htm

78. Rosa, FW., et al. "Absence of antibody response to simian virus 40 after inoculation with killed-poliovirus vaccine of mother's offspring with neurological tumors." *New*

England Journal of Medicine 1988;318:1469.

79. Rosa, FW., et al. "Response to: Neurological tumors in offspring after inoculation of mothers with killed poliovirus vaccine." *New England Journal of Medicine* 1988;319:1226.

80. See Note 47, p. 58.

81. Martini, F., et al. "SV-40 early region and large T antigen in human brain tumors, peripheral blood cells, and sperm fluids from healthy individuals." *Cancer Research* 1996;56(20): 4820–25.

82. See Note 72, p. 163.

83. See Note 81.

84. See Note 74, pp. 10 and 13.

85. National Cancer Institute (June 2001). See Note 74, p.11.

86. Koprowski, H. In a letter sent to the Congressional Health and Safety Subcommittee, April 14, 1961.

87. See Note 72, p. 159.

88. Ibid.

89. Ibid.

90. Curtis, T. "Expert says test vaccine: backs check of polio stocks for AIDS virus." *The Houston Post* (March 22, 1992):A21.

91. Ibid. Also see Note 74, p. 5.

92. Essex, M., et al. "The origin of the AIDS virus." *Scientific American* 1988; 259:64–71.

93. Karpas, A. "Origin and spread of AIDS." *Nature* 1990;348:578.

94. Kyle, WS. "Simian retroviruses, poliovaccine, and origin of AIDS." *Lancet* 1992; 339:600–1.

95. Elswood, BF., Stricker, RB. "Polio vaccines and the origin of AIDS." *Medical Hypothesis* 1994:42:347–54.

96. Myers, G, et al. "The emergence of simian/human immunodeficiency viruses." *AIDS Research and Human Retroviruses* 1992:8: 373–86.

97. "Workshop on simian virus-40 (SV-40): A possible human polyomavirus." *National Vaccine Information Center* (January 27-28, 1997). Includes a summary of evidence presented at the Eighth Annual Houston Conference on AIDS.

98. Martin, B. "Polio vaccines and the origin of AIDS: the career of a threatening idea." *Townsend Letter for Doctors* (January 1994):97–100.

99. Curtis, T. "Did a polio vaccine experiment unleash AIDS in Africa?" *The Washington Post* (April 5, 1992):C3+.

100. See Note 47, pp. 54+.

101. See Note 90 and Notes 92-95.

102. World Health Organization. "T-lymphotropic retroviruses of nonhuman primates. WHO informal meeting." *Weekly Epidemiology Records* 1985;30:269–70.

103. Curtis, T. "The origin of AIDS: A startling new theory attempts to answer the question 'Was it an act of God or an act of man?'" *Rolling Stone* (March 19, 1992):54+.

104. See Note 95.

105. See Notes 93 and 95.

106. Ohta, Y., et al. "No evidence for the contamination of live oral poliomyelitis vaccines with simian immunodeficiency virus." *AIDS* 1989;3:183–5.

107. Huet, T., et al. "Genetic organization of a chimpanzee lentivirus related to HIV-1." *Nature* 1990;345:356–9.

108. Desrosiers, RC. "HIV-1 origins: A finger on the missing link." *Nature* 1990;345:288–9.

109. Sabin, AB. "Properties and behavior of orally administered attenuated polio-virus vaccine." *Journal of the American Medical Association* 1957;164: 1216–23.

110. Plotkin, SA., Koprowski, H., et al. "Clinical trials in infants of orally administered poliomyelitis viruses." *Pediatrics* 1959;23:1041–62.

111. Barin, F., et al. "Serological evidence for virus related to simian T-lymphotropic

retrovirus III in residents of West Africa." *The Lancet* 1985;ii:1387–9.

112. See Note 103, pp. 106+.

113. See Note 72, p. 161.

114. Rustigan, R., et al. "Infection of monkey kidney tissue cultures with virus-like agents." *Proc. of the Society for Exp. Biology and Medicine* 1955;88: 8–16.

115. See Note 98, p. 100.

116. Morris, JA., et al. "Recovery of cytopathogenic agent from chimpanzees with coryza (22538). *Proceedings of the Society for Experimental Biology and Medicine* 1956;92:544–9.

117. Scheibner, V. *Vaccination: 100 Years of Orthodox Research Shows that Vaccines Represent a Medical Assault on the Immune System.* (Blackheath, NSW, Australia: Scheibner Publications, 1993):153.

118. Martin, J., et al. "African green monkey origin of the atypical cytopathic 'stealth virus' isolated from a patient with chronic fatigue syndrome." *Clinical and Diagnostic Virology* 1995;4:93–103.

119. Fisher, B. "Microbiologist issues a challenge to science: did the first oral polio vaccine lots contaminated with monkey viruses create a monkey-human hybrid called HIV-1?" *The Vaccine Reaction* (April 1996):3.

120. Eighth Annual Houston Conference on AIDS in America, 1996.

121. *American Journal of Hygiene* 1958;68:31–44.

122. See Note 119, p. 1.

123. Pallansch, MA., et al. "The eradication of polio—progress and challenges." *New England Journal of Medicine* (December 14, 2006);355(24):2508-2511.

124. Ibid.

125. Ibid.

126. See Note 3.

127. Fisher, B. "Vaccine safety consumer group cites conflict of interest in government report on cancer and contaminated polio vaccine link." *National Vaccine Information Center (NVIC); Press Release* (January 27, 1998).

128. Associated Press. "Monkey virus stirs debate: should animals be used to produce vaccines?" *CNN Interactive* (January 29, 1997).

129. Ibid.

130. See Note 76.

131. Institute of Medicine. *Vaccine Safety Forum Workshop* (November 1995).

132. See Note 119, pp. 4-5 and Note 120.

133. Ibid.

Influenza (Flu)

What is influenza?
Influenza, or the flu, is a contagious respiratory infection caused by a virus. It usually strikes during winter. Symptoms include fever, chills, runny nose, sore throat, cough, headache, muscle aches, fatigue, and decreased appetite. Conditions usually improve in two to three days. Treatment mainly consists of allowing the disease to run its course. Antibiotics will not subdue the flu virus. Bed rest and drinking lots of fluids are often recommended.

How dangerous is the flu?
The flu can lead to complications, such as pneumonia, in high risk groups. People who are at greater risk of complications from the flu mainly include the elderly and other people with preexisting medical problems, such as heart, lung, or kidney dysfunctions. People with diabetes, anemia, or compromised immune systems are also at greater risk of complications from influenza. In some instances, severe complications in high risk groups can lead to death.

How prevalent is the flu?
Every year, thousands of people contract the flu. It is a common ailment because there are three main types of flu virus, and each type can mutate, or change, from year to year. This makes it difficult to develop immunity to the disease.

The flu vaccine:
Each year, in January or February, authorities travel overseas to assess the composition of currently circulating flu viruses. They expect these same viruses to arrive in the United States several months later, in October or November (at the beginning of the flu season), causing many people to catch the flu. Thus, as soon as the authorities determine which flu viruses are anticipated to circulate in the U.S. later that year, they instruct flu vaccine manufacturers to include those strains in their products. For example, during the 2010-2011 flu season, flu vaccines were required to contain A/California/7/2009 (H1N1); A/Perth/16/2009 (H3N2); and B/Brisbane/60/2008. (Because the flu is caused by several influenza viruses, they have been classified into types A, B, and C, and further classified into subtypes with names of cities, states or countries.)

In the United States, five injectable flu vaccines produced by separate manufacturers are currently licensed for use. The FDA also approved a live-virus nasal spray vaccine that is squirted up the nose. Although each vaccine is indicated for different age groups, and may be made with different ingredients, they all contain the same attenuated flu viruses.

- Fluzone—Made from influenza viruses "propagated in embryonated chicken eggs" and inactivated with formaldehyde. Other ingredients include sodium phosphate, sodium chloride, polyethylene glycol p-isooctylphenyl ether, (Triton X-100), sucrose, and gelatin. Each 0.5 ml dose (from the multi-dose vial) also contains 25 mcg of mercury. Produced by Sanofi Pasteur. Indicated for individuals 6 months of age and older.[1]
- FluMist—A live-virus nasal spray vaccine. Made by inoculating eggs "with each of the reassortant strains and incubated to allow vaccine virus replication." Ingredients include sucrose, potassium phosphate, monosodium phosphate, monosodium glutamate (MSG), gentamicin sulfate, hydrolyzed porcine gelatin (from pigs), and ethylene diamine tetracetic acid. Produced by MedImmune. Indicated for individuals 2 to 49 years of age.[2]
- Fluvirin—Ingredients include neomycin, polymyxin, nonylphenol ethoxylate, betapropiolactone, and "residual amounts of egg proteins." Each 0.5 ml dose (from the multi-dose vial) also contains 25 mcg of mercury. Produced by Novartis. Indicated for individuals 4 years of age and older.[3]

Some brands of the flu vaccine are only indicated for adults 18 years of age and older:
- Afluria—Ingredients include sodium chloride, sodium phosphate, potassium chloride, potassium phosphate, calcium chloride, sodium taurodeoxycholate, ovalbumin, neomycin, polymyxin B, and beta-propiolactone. Each 0.5 ml dose (from the multi-dose vial) also contains 24.5 mcg of mercury. Produced by CSL Biotherapies.[4]
- Fluarix—Ingredients include sucrose, sodium chloride, sodium phosphate, sodium deoxycholate, ovalbumin (residual egg proteins), octoxynol-10 (Triton X-100), polysorbate 80 (Tween 80), gentamicin sulfate, a-tocopheryl hydrogen succinate, hydrocortisone, and formaldehyde. Produced by GSK.[5]
- Flulaval—Each dose contains sodium deoxycholate, formaldehyde, residual egg proteins, and 25 mcg of mercury. Produced by GSK.[6]

Can the Flu Vaccine Cause the Flu?

Common reactions to the flu vaccine include flu-like symptoms which can last several days: fever, chills, sore throat, runny nose, nasal congestion, headache, muscle aches, abdominal pain, and fatigue. Physicians often claim that it's not possible to contract the flu from the flu vaccine. However, this contradicts the real-life experiences of many people. Besides, vaccines are designed to stimulate the immune system by mimicking disease. This has been openly acknowledged by some authorities. For example, according to Chris Anna Mink, MD, a medical officer with the FDA, "because [FluMist] is live, it can grow in the nose and some people get flu symptoms...."[7] Other authorities concede that in people with weak immune systems, "the vaccine virus can reproduce and create live virus which can cause flu symptoms and even the flu."[8]

The following comments are typical of people who were vaccinated against flu yet still caught the disease:

"I've had the flu vaccine twice, and on both occasions I had the worst case of flu in my entire life. Never, ever again. Waste of time and money."

"I was required to take a flu shot when I was in the army and I woke up the next morning sick as a dog. As a result, I didn't take a flu shot until recently when my doctor recommended it after I got pneumonia. I still caught the flu."[9]

Safety

Serious reactions to the flu vaccine include life-threatening allergies to vaccine components, and **Guillain-Barré syndrome** (GBS), a severe paralytic disease. GBS can occur several weeks following a flu vaccine and is fatal in about one of every 20 victims.[10] In addition to GBS, numerous studies have investigated and/or documented other serious adverse reactions to the flu vaccine, causing severe disorders that affect the immune, nervous, respiratory, skin, blood, and lymphatic systems. Flu vaccine manufacturers acknowledge that many of these ailments occurred after flu vaccinations. These include: convulsions, myelitis, Bell's palsy, Stevens-Johnson syndrome, encephalopathy, myasthenia, facial paralysis, neuropathy, optic neuritis, paresthesia, thrombocytopenia, lymphadenopathy, reactive arthritis, arthralgia, myalgia, wheezing, difficulty breathing, and "asthmatic exacerbations" in persons with a history of asthma.[11-48]

Flu Scare Tactics and
Vaccine Marketing Strategies

Every year, just prior to the impending flu season, the CDC asserts that 36,000 people die *annually* from the flu. However, according to the CDC's own official records documented in *National Vital Statistics Reports,* only a few hundred people die from influenza on an average year. For example, in 2003, 1,792 people died from the flu. In 2002, 727 people died from the flu. The year before that, in 2001, just 257 people died from the flu.[49] Many of these deaths occurred in people with preexisting medical conditions.

In April 2004, the CDC sponsored a confidential vaccine summit for leaders of health institutions, vaccine manufacturers, and select media organizations. The purpose of this private gathering was to "Foster Higher Interest and Demand for Influenza Vaccine."[50] Participants were taught how to frighten the public into obtaining flu vaccine at any cost. For example, public health authorities were urged to "predict dire outcomes" prior to the flu season. Communication directors were shown how to increase anxiety by publishing "desirable phrases" in the media, emphasizing "very severe" and "deadly" strains of flu.[51]

In October 2005, the *British Medical Journal (BMJ)* published a special report criticizing the CDC's marketing campaign of fear in which medical experts are taught to irrationally scare people to raise demand for flu vaccine. Data culled from the CDC's own official records was presented, confirming that the CDC intentionally hyperinflates influenza mortality numbers to alarm the public and increase flu vaccine sales. *BMJ* acknowledged that CDC flu deaths are concocted for "public relations" rather than determined by science.[52]

Influenza vaccine safety in children:

In February 2005, *The Lancet* published a review of all pertinent influenza vaccine studies in children and found "clear evidence of systematic suppression of safety data." For example, authors of the original studies were denied access to safety data from their own clinical trials. In one influenza vaccine study, vaccinated children had nearly twice as many "medical adverse events" as unvaccinated children. However, these "events" were not adequately identified. When the vaccine manufacturer was contacted for the missing data, researchers were denied access to it because it is considered proprietary information. In addition, the CDC refuses to warn parents that safety data is lacking.[53,54]

A major influenza vaccine manufacturer, MedImmune, recently submitted a confidential document to the FDA containing safety data from studies that it conducted on its own vaccine.[55] The company was seeking permission to vaccinate children under 5 years of age with its live-virus nasal spray

FluMist vaccine (the one that is squirted up the nose). When this vaccine was originally licensed in 2003, the FDA only permitted it to be given to children 5 years of age and older because a large study conducted in 31 clinics showed that it caused "a statistically significant increase in asthma or reactive airways disease" in children under 5 years of age.[56] Nevertheless, in September 2007, the FDA licensed this vaccine for children as young as two years of age.

The flu vaccine is potentially dangerous in older children as well. For example, Maurice Lamkin, a healthy 5-year-old boy, recently received a flu shot. He ran a fever that evening and two days later had his first seizure. He was rushed to the hospital where he remained for the next 40 days fighting for his life with brain swelling. Dr. Kenneth Mack, a Mayo Clinic child neurologist who consulted on the case, said an adverse reaction to the flu vaccine can cause encephalitis: "The body's immune system can get overactive and attack the brain."[57] Maurice's doctor thinks that the flu shot was "the most likely culprit."[58] Maurice is now home but has to wear diapers and can no longer speak. According to his mother...

"He was a healthy boy, running around. He was so proud because he had just learned to read and write. He was living his life, singing, dancing, wrestling with his brother. He was perfectly fine before the flu shot."[59]
—Distraught mother of a flu-vaccinated child

Influenza mortality in children:

In 1999, before flu vaccines were recommended and given to small boys and girls, just 25 children in the United States under 5 years of age died from influenza. In 2000, 2001 and 2002, there were just 19, 13 and 12 influenza deaths, respectively, in this age group. However, in the latter half of 2002 the CDC began advocating that all young children receive flu vaccines. Thus, doctors started vaccinating as many young children as possible against the flu. The following year, in 2003, influenza deaths in children under 5 years of age skyrocketed to 90 cases—a sevenfold increase over previous years.[60,61]

VAERS: The federal government maintains a database of suspected cases of vaccine-related morbidity and mortality (side effects and death). The case reports on the following page were taken directly from the FDA's Vaccine Adverse Event Reporting System (VAERS).[62] They are just a small sample of the potential harm associated with flu vaccines. A couple of firsthand case reports by parents are included as well.[63]

Flu Vaccine: VAERS Case Reports

‣298905: A 6-month-old boy received a flu shot and collapsed while eating breakfast the next day. He was rushed to the hospital and pronounced dead.

‣330148: A 10-month-old boy received a flu shot and died the next day.

‣246080: A 14-month-old girl received a flu vaccine, developed a fever and bronchitis, and died in her sleep 2 days later.

‣295195: A 16-month-old girl received a flu shot and died the next day.

‣270156: A 1½-year-old girl receive a flu vaccine, developed a cough, fever, pneumonitis, and died 2 days later.

‣232179: A 20-month-old boy received a flu vaccine and was found "dead in the early morning about 16-20 hours after the flu vaccine." The autopsy report stated SIDS.

‣295043: A 2-year-old boy received a flu shot and died 2 hours later.

‣245502: A 2-year-old boy received a flu vaccine, developed an upper respiratory tract infection, and was "found dead in bed the following morning."

‣269826: A 2-year-old boy received a flu shot, developed viral pneumonia, went into a coma, and was pronounced dead from "cardi-respiratory arrest" two days later.

‣326590: A 2-year-old girl received the live-virus FluMist vaccine and five days later developed "sudden onset flaccid quadriplegia" (paralysis of all four limbs). Respiratory failure required intubation and a tracheostomy. The child spent 34 days in the hospital.

‣297055: A 3-year-old girl received a flu shot in the morning and by that evening she was coughing, wheezing and struggling to breathe. She spent three days in intensive care, and needed breathing treatments for another week after being discharged.

‣265978: Two hours after a flu vaccine, a 3-year-old girl developed nausea, vomiting, diarrhea, and lethargy. Over the next several days her speech got worse and she lost the ability to walk or control her bowels and urine. She was diagnosed with acute disseminated encephalomyelitis and was hospitalized.

‣336786: A 5-year-old boy received the live-virus FluMist vaccine and 17 days later was diagnosed with juvenile onset diabetes mellitus.

Case Reports by Parents

‣ *"My 2½ year-old daughter received a flu shot on a Thursday. The following Monday, I brought her back to the doctor because her eyes were suddenly crossed. The doctor sent her to ER where she was diagnosed with GBS (Guillain-Barré syndrome) from the flu shot."*

‣ *"In October, my 9-year-old daughter got her flu vaccine (nose spray) for the first time. Two days later, she started getting a terrible cold, bad headache and sick stomach. That night, she woke up with a seizure. Six days later, she had another seizure. She is now on seizure medication."*

Efficacy

Precise flu vaccine efficacy rates are difficult to ascertain and unreliable because flu strains change all the time. According to the CDC...

"Overall vaccine effectiveness varies from year to year, depending upon the degree of similarity between influenza virus strains included in the vaccine and the strain or strains that circulate during the influenza season."[64]

—**Centers for Disease Control and Prevention (CDC)**

Even when there is a good match between the viral strains comprising a flu vaccine and that year's circulating flu virus, immunity from the shot is short-lived because antibody levels begin to decline within months, and are often low one year after vaccination. Permanent immunity to a particular strain of flu is only possible by contracting the disease naturally. When natural infection is suppressed by force-vaccinating the whole population, healthy children and adults—who rarely suffer complications from flu—will not be able to develop natural antibodies and permanent immunity to that flu strain. In addition, respiratory ailments that are not caused by influenza, and disease conditions caused by flu viruses not included in the vaccine, or by microorganisms associated with different diseases, such as colds, will not be alleviated by getting an annual flu shot. Each flu vaccine is only designed to protect against the three viral strains which are included in that year's flu vaccine.

Flu vaccine efficacy in children:

The United States and Canada recently recommended influenza vaccines for healthy children as young as six months old. To assess the merits of this policy, researchers analyzed all significant influenza vaccine studies throughout the world. In February 2005, *The Lancet* published the results of their analysis. Researchers found no evidence that influenza vaccines prevent flu in children younger than 2 years old. In addition, there was "no convincing evidence that [flu] vaccines can reduce mortality, hospital admissions, serious complications and community transmission of influenza." There was also little evidence that flu vaccines could reduce secondary cases, lower respiratory tract disease or acute otitis media. According to the lead researcher, "immunization of very young children is not lent support by our findings."[65,66]

In 2006, researchers working for *The Cochrane Collaboration*—an objective, independent well-respected source of scientific evidence—analyzed all relevant influenza vaccine trials conducted on children worldwide, totaling 51 studies involving more than 260,000 children. They determined that in healthy children older than two years of age, the live flu vaccine was just 33 percent effective; the inactivated influenza vaccine was just 36 percent effective. In healthy children under two years of age, the efficacy of the inactivated flu vaccine "was similar to placebo."[67] The lead author of the review, Dr. Tom Jefferson, expressed his concern regarding American influenza vaccine policies:

> *"We just cannot understand how you can vaccinate millions of small children in the absence of convincing scientific evidence that the vaccines make any difference."*[68]
> —**Dr. Tom Jefferson, lead author of a major flu vaccine study**

In October 2008, *Archives of Pediatrics and Adolescent Medicine* published a study that analyzed influenza vaccine effectiveness in children aged 6 months to 5 years. The study was conducted over two consecutive flu seasons. Authors of the study "could not demonstrate vaccine effectiveness" at reducing influenza-related doctor or hospital visits.[69]

Flu vaccine efficacy in healthy adults:
Independent researchers working for *The Cochrane Collaboration* reviewed the evidence of influenza vaccine efficacy in healthy adults. They analyzed 25 studies involving thousands of people and discovered that in healthy adults under 65 years of age, influenza vaccination "did not affect hospital stay, time off from work, or death from influenza and its complications." Authors of the study concluded that "universal immunization of healthy adults is not supported" by the data.[70]

Flu vaccine efficacy in the elderly:
Influenza vaccination of the elderly is recommended worldwide. To assess this policy, independent researchers working for *The Cochrane Collaboration* conducted a thorough, systematic review of 64 studies carried out over 40 years of influenza vaccinations. Their results showed that for the elderly living in the community, influenza vaccines "were not significantly effective against influenza or pneumonia." For the elderly living in group homes—*in years when the vaccine is a good match with the circulating influenza virus*—the influenza vaccine is merely 23 percent

effective against "influenza-like illness," 46 percent effective against pneumonia, and "non-significant against influenza." Researchers found no correlation between the percentage of people vaccinated and the overall rate of influenza-like illness.[71]

Vaccine failures in the elderly are typical—even when there is a precise match between the flu vaccine strain and the current flu virus. For example, in one flu outbreak in a Minnesota nursing home, 95 percent of the residents, and 72 percent of the staff members with direct patient contact had been vaccinated 4 to 8 weeks prior to the outbreak. Authorities were baffled when they discovered that the viral strain isolated from the outbreak was "antigenically identical" to the one in the vaccine. In other words, the vaccine was a "perfect" match for that year's circulating flu virus yet it was a complete failure. The authors of the study concluded that "despite widespread vaccination...influenza outbreaks continue to occur."[72]

In February 2005, the *Archives of Internal Medicine* published a comprehensive study that analyzed immunization data from 33 influenza seasons, from 1968 through 2001. In the United States, just 15 percent of elderly persons were vaccinated before 1980. By 2001, 65 percent were vaccinated, yet influenza-related mortality actually *increased* during this period. In other words, although immunization rates in people 65 years or older increased by 50 percentage points during a 20-year period, there has not been a corresponding decline in flu (or pneumonia) related deaths. According to the authors of the study...

> *"We could not correlate increasing [flu] vaccination coverage...with declining mortality rates in any age group. We conclude that observational studies substantially overestimate vaccination benefit."*[73]
> **—Archives of Internal Medicine**

In February 2010, impartial scientists concluded that "the available evidence is of poor quality and provides no guidance regarding the safety...or effectiveness of influenza vaccines for people aged 65 years or older."[74]

Flu vaccine efficacy in healthcare workers:

Healthcare workers (nurses, hospital workers, etc.) are often required to receive annual flu vaccines because authorities are concerned that they might transmit influenza to those in their care, especially the elderly. To assess the merits of this policy, researchers working for *The Cochrane Collaboration* reviewed all pertinent studies and discovered that staff vaccinations "have no efficacy against influenza." They concluded:

"There is no...evidence that vaccinating healthcare workers reduces the incidence of influenza or its complications in the elderly in institutions.... An incremental benefit of vaccinating healthcare workers for the benefit of the elderly cannot be proven."[75] —**The Cochrane Collaboration**

In February 2010, independent scientists once again concluded that "vaccinating healthcare workers who look after the elderly in long-term care facilities did not show any effect on...laboratory-proven influenza, pneumonia or deaths from pneumonia."[76]

Additional influenza vaccine efficacy studies:

In October 2006, the *British Medical Journal* published a paper that analyzed all pertinent influenza vaccination studies and concluded there is a large gap between evidence of the flu vaccine's efficacy and the influenza policies established by health agencies. According to the author of the paper, Dr. Tom Jefferson, "Every year enormous effort goes into producing influenza vaccines for that specific year and delivering them to appropriate sections of the population. Is this effort justified?"[77] Apparently not. Flu vaccines had little or no effect on influenza campaign objectives, such as hospital stay, time off work, or death from influenza and its complications. Flu vaccines were found to be ineffective in children under 2 years of age, in healthy adults under 65 years of age, and in people 65 years and older. There is little evidence that flu vaccines are beneficial when given to healthcare workers to protect their patients, when given to children to reduce transmission of the virus to family contacts, or when given to vulnerable people, such as those with asthma and cystic fibrosis.[78-82] Jefferson found little proof of the flu vaccine's merit: "There is a misfit between the evidence and policy, and taxpayers ought to ask why."[83]

In December 2006, the *New England Journal of Medicine* published a study on vaccinating all school children to reduce the spread of flu in communities. Researchers wanted to determine whether vaccinating one group of people—children—would provide "herd immunity" for, or protect, another group of people—their families and neighbors. They vaccinated children in some schools (intervention schools) but not in others (control-group schools), then tallied the rates of absenteeism, illness and hospitalizations. The results surprised the investigators: Although there were fewer "influenza-like symptoms" in households with children in the intervention schools than in households with children in the control-group schools, *intervention school households (both children and adults) had significantly higher rates of hospitalization.* There were no differences in missed days of school. In addition, children who received the flu vaccine had a "statistically significant increase in influenza-like symptoms" after vaccination. They also took more drugs to control undesirable side effects.[84]

In December 2009, *The Lancet* published a study showing that annual flu shots prevent immunity to future strains of the disease. Children who are vaccinated every year against seasonal flu may be *more* susceptible to dangerous pandemic strains than are children that get seasonal flu.[85] In a study of mice vaccinated against seasonal flu strains, they developed severe disease and died when exposed to alternate strains. Unvaccinated mice became less ill and did not die when exposed to more lethal strains.[86]

Are annual flu shots recommended?

The CDC and vaccine industry wish to vaccinate more and more people against influenza. Initially, the CDC strongly encouraged the elderly—people over 65 years of age—to receive annual flu shots. Then authorities lowered the recommended age to 50. Soon thereafter, all nursing home residents, staff members and healthcare workers were expected to receive annual flu shots. Next, the CDC added pregnant women to the list—*even though flu shots contain mercury and the CDC admits that pregnant women and their fetuses are highly vulnerable to mercury.*[87] (Pregnancy was initially a contraindication to the flu shot before the CDC altered its own advice.)[88]

In 2004, the CDC recommended that children aged 6 to 23 months, receive annual flu vaccines. In 2006, the CDC expanded its recommendations to include children up to 59 months of age, and also added household contacts of children, and caregivers of young children, to the list of people expected to receive annual flu shots. In 2008, the list was expanded again to include children and teenagers up to age 18. In 2010, the CDC declared that *all* people aged 6 months and older should get annual flu vaccinations.

Do doctors and healthcare workers get annual flu shots?

In the Fall of 2005, the Johns Hopkins University initiated a campaign to mandate influenza vaccination for all healthcare workers. However, despite free and easy access to the vaccine, only 40 percent voluntarily get one; 30 percent are afraid of catching the flu from the vaccine itself.[89] In a nationally representative study of 1,651 U.S. healthcare workers (e.g., nurses aides and medical assistants), researchers at Harvard University and the University of Southern California discovered that 62 percent were *not* vaccinated against the flu.[90] A survey reported by the *Associated Press* found that doctors and nurses are among the *least* likely to be vaccinated. In fact, 70 percent of doctors and nurses do *not* get annual flu shots.[91]

Avian flu:

In April of 2007 the FDA approved for human use, a bird flu vaccine, "despite concerns it might not be that effective at protecting people against avian influenza."[92] The vaccine is being stockpiled by the U.S. government in case the bird flu virus mutates and rapidly spreads among people.

Swine flu:

Swine flu is similar to the seasonal flu. The virus is spread when infected people cough or sneeze. Symptoms include a fever, headache, sore throat, aches and chills. Vomiting and diarrhea may occur as well. In April 2009, a new strain of swine flu—novel influenza A (H1N1) infection—was detected. It contained a unique mix of genetic material from human, bird, and pig viruses. The infection was passed from person to person around the world. Although most people who became ill recovered without requiring medical treatment, on June 11, 2009 the World Health Organization declared a pandemic due to the rapid spread of the virus.

Although swine flu can be treated with antiviral medicine, authorities initiated a campaign to develop several new swine flu vaccines and vaccinate the population. This also occurred in 1976, when the CDC made up a false tale of deadly swine flu epidemics sweeping the nation if mass vaccinations were not instituted. U.S. citizens were systematically vaccinated, and several weeks later hundreds were stricken with the crippling Guillain-Barré syndrome; several of the vaccinated people died.[93,94]

Vitamin D and influenza:

Researchers have known for many years that influenza mainly occurs in the winter when there is less sun, and is less prevalent near the equator where there is lots of sun. Today, we also know that when people are exposed to ultraviolet radiation (from sunlight or artificial sources) they produce vitamin D. Vitamin D deficiency is relatively common. In a landmark study published in *Epidemiology and Infection,* researchers linked these pieces of the puzzle together and showed that vitamin D deficiency weakens the immune system creating susceptibility to influenza. Vitamin D supplements (2000-4000 i.u. daily)—especially in the winter—may provide protective benefits against the flu.[95-97]

In June of 2009, Wisconsin experienced an increase in cases of swine flu (H1N1). At Central Wisconsin Center (CWC), a long-term care facility for people with developmental disabilities, 60 of the 800 staff members (7.5 percent) developed influenza-like illness or were documented to have swine flu. In contrast, only two of the 275 residents (0.73 percent) developed influenza-like illness. This 10-fold difference is statistically significant. Dr. Norris Glick, a medical doctor at CWC, provides a likely explanation: "Serum 25-OHD (a measure of vitamin D in the blood) has been monitored in virtually all residents for several years and patients supplemented with vitamin D."[98] (Staff members were not given vitamin D supplements.) According to vitamin D expert, Dr. John Cannell:

> *"The is the first hard data that I am aware of concerning [swine flu] and vitamin D. It appears that vitamin D is protective against H1N1."*[99]
> —**John Cannell, MD, vitamin D expert**

Dr. Ellie Campbell made similar observations at her medical practice in Georgia. She regularly measures vitamin D levels in her patients and supplements them with vitamin D (2,000-5,000 i.u.). She shares an office with another family physician who does not give vitamin D to his patients. He is seeing up to 10 cases of influenza-like illness every week. Dr. Campbell has had no cases.[100]

These examples provide strong evidence that vitamin D protects against influenza. In addition, a large study published in the July-August 2009 issue of *Endocrine Practice* found compelling evidence supporting further research into using vitamin D to not just prevent, but to *treat* influenza and upper respiratory tract illnesses.[101] I consider the "sunshine vitamin" to be an inexpensive insurance policy. (For more information about the potential benefits of vitamin D, turn to page 130 in the chapter on autism.)

Notes

1. Sanofi Pasteur. "Influenza virus vaccine, Fluzone" (June 2008).
2. MedImmune. "FluMist, influenza virus vaccine live" (June 2008).
3. Novartis. "Influenza virus vaccine, Fluvirin" (July 2008).
4. CSL, Ltd. "Afluria, influenza virus vaccine" (2007).
5. GlaxoSmithKline. "Influenza virus vaccine, Fluarix" (July 2009).
6. GlaxoSmithKline. "Flulaval (influenza virus vaccine)" (2009).
7. Meadows, M. *FDA Consumer Magazine* (Sept-Oct. 2003).
8. "What's up with FluMist?" *Hlth Serv Columbia U.* 2010. www.goaskalice.columbia.edu
9. "Flu vaccines 'not worth the bother' says expert." *Mail Online* (October 2006). www.dailymail.co.uk
10. National Vaccine Information Center (NVIC). "The flu and the flu vaccine." www.909shot.com
11. Lohse, A., et al. "Vascular purpura and cryoglobulinemia after influenza vaccination. Case-report and literature review." *Rev Rhum Engl Ed.* (June 1999); 66(6):359-60.
12. Schmutz, JL, et al. "Does influenza vaccination induce bullous pemphigoid?" *Ann Dermatol Vernereol.* (October 1999);126(10):765. [French.]
13. Cummins, D., et al. "Haematological changes associated with influenza vaccination in people aged over 65: case report and prospective study." *Clin Lab Haematol* (Oct 1998);20(5):285-7.

46 Make an Informed Vaccine Decision

14. Downs, AM., et al. "Does influenza vaccination induce bullous pemphigoid? A report of four cases." *Br J Dermatol* (February 1998);138(2):363.
15. Kawasaki, A., et al. "Bilateral anterior ischemic optic neuropathy following influenza vaccination." *J Neuroophthalmol* (March 1998);18(1):56-9.
16. Lasky, T., et al. "The Guillain-Barré syndrome and the 1992-1993 and 1993-1994 influenza vaccines." *N Engl J Med* (December 1998);339(25):1797-802.
17. Park, CL, et al. "Does influenza vaccination exacerbate asthma?" *Drug Saf.* (August 1998);19(2):83-8.
18. Ramakrishnan, N, et al. "Thrombotic thrombocytopenic purpura following influenza vaccination—a brief case report." *Conn Med.* (Oct. 1998);62(10):587-8.
19. Selvaraj, N., et al. "Hemiparesis following influenza vaccination." *Postgrad Med J.* (October 1998);74(876):633-5.
20. Confino, I., et al. "Erythromelalgia following influenza vaccine in a child." *Clin Exp Rheumatol* (Jan-Feb 1997);15(1): 111-3.
21. Desson, JF., et al. "Acute benign pericarditis after anti-influenza vaccination." *Presse Med.* (March 22, 1997);26(9):415. [French.]
22. Hull, TP., et al. "Optic neuritis after influenza vaccination." *Am J Ophthalmol* (Nov1997);124(5):703-4.
23. Kelsall, JT., et al. "Microscopic polyangitis after influenza vaccination." *J Rheumatol.* (June 1997);24(6):1198-1202.
24. Owensby, JE., et al. "Cellulitis and myositis caused by Agrobacterium radiobacter and Haemophilus parainfluenzae after influenza virus vaccination." *South Med J.* (July 1997);90(7):752-4.
25. Bernad Valles, M., et al. "Adverse reactions to different types of influenza vaccines." *Med Clin (Barc)* (January 13, 1996);106(1):11-4. [Spanish.]
26. Fournier, B., et al. "Bullous pemphigoid induced by vaccination." *Br J Dermatol.* (July 1996);135(1):153-4.
27. Honkanen, PO., et al. "Reactions following administration of influenza vaccine along with pneumococcal vaccine to the elderly." *Arch Int Med* (Jan 22, 1996);156(2):205-8.
28. Lear, JT., et al. "Bullous pemphigoid following influenza vaccination." *Clin Exp Dermatol.* (Sep 1996); 21(5):392.
29. Ray, CL., et al. "Bilateral optic neuropathy associated with influenza vaccination." *J Neuroophthalmol.* (Sep 1996); 16(3):182-4.
30. Antony, SJ., et al. "Postvaccinial (influenza) disseminated encephalopathy (Brown-Sequard syndrome)." *J Natl Med Assoc* (Sep 1995);87(9):705-8.
31. Cambiaghi, S., et al. "Gianotti-Crosti syndrome in an adult after influenza virus vaccination." *Dermatology* 1995; 191(4):340-1.
32. Herderschee, D., et al. "Myelopathy following influenza vaccination." *Ned Tijdschr Geneeskd* (October 21, 1995); 139(42):2152-4. [Dutch.]
33. Biasi, D., et al. "A case of reactive arthritis after influenza after influenza vaccination." *Clin Rheumatol* (December 1994); 13(4)645.
34. Blanche, P., et al. "Development of uveitis following vaccination for influenza." *Clin Infect Dis* (November 1994); 19(5):979.
35. Bodokh, I., et al. "Reactivation of bullous pemphigoid after influenza vaccination." *Therapie.* (Mar-Apr 1994);49(2): 154. [French.]
36. Brown, MA., et al. "Rheumatic complications of influenza vaccination." *Aust N Z J Med.* (October 1994); 24(5):572-3.
37. Beijer, WE., et al. "Polymyalgia rheumatica and influenza vaccination." *Dtsch Med Wochenschr.* (February 5, 1993);118(5): 164-5. [German.]
38. Boutros, N., et al. "Delirium following influenza vaccination." *Am J Psychiatry.* (Dec 1993);150(12):1899.
39. Mader, R., et al. "Systemic vasculitis following influenza vaccination —report of 3 cases and literature review." *J Rheumatol* (August 1993);20(8):1429-31.
40. Robinson, T., et al. "Side effects of influenza vaccination." *Br J Gen Pract.* (Nov 1992);42(364):489-90.
41. Ward, DL. Re: "Guillian-Barré syndrome and influenza vaccination in the US Army, 1980-1988." *Am J Epidemiol* (August 1, 1992);136(3):374-6.

42. Young, G. "Side effects of influenza immunization." *Br J Gen Pract* (March 1992);42(356):131.
43. Roscelli, JD., et al. "Guillain-Barré syndrome and influenza vaccination in the US Army, 1980-1988." *Am J Epidemiol* (May 1, 1991);133(9):952-5.
44. Molina, M., et al. "Leukocytoclastic vasculitis secondary to flu vaccination." *Med Clin (Barc).* (June 9, 1990);95(2):78. [Spanish.]
45. Pelosio, A., et al. "Influenza vaccination and poly-radiculoneuritis of the Guillain-Barré type." *Medicina (Firenze)* (Apr-Jun 1990);10(2):169. [Italian.]
46. Buchner, H., et al. "Polyneuritis cranialis? Brain stem encephalitis and myelitis after preventive influenza vaccination." *Nervenarzt* (Nov 1988);59(11):679-82. [German]
47. Gnanasekaran, SK., et al. "Influenza vaccination among children with asthma in Medicaid managed care." *Ambulatory Pediatrics* 2006;6:1-7.
48. See Notes 1-6.
49. CDC. "Deaths: final data..." *National Vital Statistics Reports:* 52(3); 53(5); 54(13).
50. Nowak, G. "Planning for the 2004-2005 influenza vaccination season: a communication situation analysis." *Department of Health and Human Services.*
51. Ibid.
52. Doshi, P. "Are U.S. flu death figures more PR than science?" *British Medical Journal* (December 10, 2005);331:1412.
53. Jefferson, T., et al. "Assessment of the efficacy and effectiveness of influenza vaccines in healthy children: systematic review." *The Lancet* 2005;365(Feb. 26):773-80.
54. Napoli, M. "Doubts about safety of flu vaccine in kids." *Center for Medical Consumers* (Oct 2005). medicalconsumers.org
55. FDA. "FluMist® live, attenuated influenza vaccine briefing document: prior approval supplemental BLA, indication extension to include children less than 5 years of age." (Confidential document.) *FDA Vaccines and Related Biological Products Advisory Committee* (April 19, 2007.)
56. See Note 2.
57. Dorsett, A. "Boy's illness a mystery." *Express News, San Antonio* (March 10, 2005).
58. Ibid.
59. Ibid.
60. CDC. "Deaths: final data..." *Nat Vital Stat Rep:* 49(8); 50(15); 52(3); 53(5); 54(13).
61. AAP News. "Flu vaccine extended to kids 6-23 months." *AAP* (August 2002).
62. National Vaccine Information Center. "MedAlerts: access to the U.S. government's Vaccine Adverse Event Reporting System (VAERS)." www.medalerts.org
63. Thinktwice Global Vaccine Institute. Unsolicited case reports submitted by concerned parents. www.thinktwice.com
64. CDC. "Vaccine Information: Influenza Vaccine." www.cdc.gov
65. See Note 53.
66. Roos, R. "Efficacy of flu shots in children under 2 questioned." *Center for Infectious Disease Research and Policy* (February 25, 2005).
67. Smith, S., et al. "Vaccines for preventing influenza in healthy children." *The Cochrane Collaboration: Cochrane Database of Systematic Reviews* (John Wiley & Sons, Ltd.), 2006(1). Art. No. CD004879.
68. Alliance for Human Research Protection. "Oxford study—no evidence flu vaccine works in infants: USA and Canada's influenza vaccination programmes for children based on little evidence" (February 25, 2005).
69. Szilagyi, PG., et al. "Influenza vaccine effectiveness among children 6 to 59 months of age during two influenza seasons." *Arch Pediatr Adol Med* 2008;162(10): 943-51.
70. Rivetti, D., et al. "Vaccines for preventing influenza in healthy adults." *The Cochrane Collaboration: Cochrane Database of Systematic Reviews* (John Wiley & Sons, Ltd.), 2004(3). Art. No. CD001269.
71. Rivetti, D., et al. "Vaccines for preventing influenza in the elderly." *The Cochrane Collaboration: Cochrane Database of Systematic Reviews* (John Wiley & Sons, Ltd.), 2006(3). Art. No. CD004876.
72. Kuhle, CL., et al. "An influenza outbreak in an immunized nursing home population: inadequate host response or vaccine failure?" *Annals of Long-Term Care* 1998;6[3]:72.

73. Simonsen, L., et al. "Impact of influenza vaccination on seasonal mortality in the U.S. elderly population." *Archives of Internal Medicine* 2005;165:265-72.

74. Jefferson T., et al. "Vaccines for preventing influenza in the elderly." *Cochrane Database of Systematic Reviews* 2010, Issue 2. Art. No.: CD004876.

75. Thomas, RE., et al. "Influenza vaccination for healthcare workers who work with the elderly." *The Cochrane Collaboration: Cochrane Database of Systematic Reviews* (John Wiley & Sons, Ltd.), 2006(3). Art. No. CD005187.

76. Thomas RE., et al. "Influenza vaccination for healthcare workers who work with the elderly." *Cochrane Database of Systematic Reviews* 2010, Issue 2. Art. No.: CD005187.

77. Jefferson, T. "Influenza vaccination: policy versus evidence." *BMJ* 2006; 333:912-915.

78. Ibid.

79. Cates, CJ., et al. "Vaccines for preventing influenza in people with asthma." *The Cochrane Collaboration: Cochrane Database of Systematic Reviews* (John Wiley & Sons, Ltd.), 2007(2). Art. No. CD000364.

80. Bhalla, P., et al. "Vaccines for preventing influenza in people with cystic fibrosis." *The Cochrane Collaboration: Cochrane Database of Systematic Reviews* (John Wiley & Sons, Ltd.), 2007(2). Art. No. CD001753.

81. CTV News. "Report casts doubt on flu vaccine effectiveness." (October 26, 2006).

82. BBC News. "Winter flu jab's evidence queried." (October 26, 2006).

83. Ibid.

84. King, Jr., JC., et al. "Effectiveness of school-based influenza vaccination." *New England Journal of Medicine* 2006;355:2523-32.

85. Bodewes, R., et al. "Yearly influenza vaccinations: a double-edged sword?" *The Lancet* (December 2009);9(12):784-88.

86. Bodewes R., et al. "Vaccination against human influenza A/H3N2 virus prevents the induction of heterosubtypic immunity against lethal infection with avian influenza A/H5N1 virus." *PLoS One* 2009;4(5):e5538.

87. CDC. "Frequently asked questions about mercury and thimerosal." www.cdc.gov/vaccinesafety/updates/thimerosal_faqs_mercury.htm (Last visited: August 9, 2009).

88. Fisher, BL. "Informed consent advocate says government and industry should release flu vaccine effectiveness data." Press release. *Nat Vac Information Center* (Dec 10, 2003).

89. Johns Hopkins. "Johns Hopkins flu expert calls for mandatory vaccination of healthcare workers; view is subject to debate." www.hopkinsnet.jhu.edu

90. Woolhandler, S., et al. "Brief report: influenza vaccination and health care workers in the United States." *J of General Internal Medicine* (February 6, 2006).

91. Recer, P. "Study: health workers major sources of flu in old-age homes." *Associated Press* (October 9, 1997).

92. Corbett, J. "FDA approves Sanofi-Aventis H5N1 bird-flu vaccine." *Marketwatch* (April 17, 2007).

93. Hurwitz, ES., et al. "Guillain-Barré syndrome and the 1978-79 influenza vaccine." *New England Journal of Medicine* 1981;304:1557-61.

94. Kaplan, JE., et al. "Guillain-Barré syndrome in the U.S., 1978-1981: Additional observations from the national surveillance system." *Neurology* (May 1983);33(5):633-37.

95. Cannell, JJ., et al. "Epidemic influenza and vitamin D." *Epidemiology and Infection* (December 2006);134(6):1129-40.

96. Totheroh, G. "What's the real story on vitamin D? *CBN News Science and Medical Reporter* (November 17, 2007).

97. Schor, J. "Vitamin D and influenza." *Naturopathy Digest* (October 17, 2008).

98. In a September 2009 email from Dr. Norris Glick to Dr. John Cannell, posted on the Vitamin D Council's website. www.vitamindcouncil.org

99. Cannell, J. "Vitamin D and H1N1 swine flu." *The Vitamin D Newsletter, Special Report* (September 2009). www.vitamindcouncil.org

100. In a September 2009 email from Dr. Ellie Campbell to Dr. John Cannell, posted on the Vitamin D Council's website. www.vitamindcouncil.org

101. Yamshchikov, AV., et al. "Vitamin D for treatment and prevention of infectious diseases: a systematic review of randomized controlled trials." *Endocr Pract* (July-August 2009);15(5):438-49.

Tetanus

What is tetanus?

Tetanus is a non-contagious bacterial disease that causes severe muscular contractions. It is also called *lockjaw* because some victims are unable to open their mouths or swallow. Other symptoms include depression, headaches, and spasms that interfere with breathing.

Tetanus is caused by toxins produced by a bacterium called *Clostridium tetani*. The dormant spores live in soil, dust, and manure. They can enter the body through cuts and puncture wounds, but will only multiply in an anaerobic (oxygen-free) environment. The incubation period, from the time of the injury until the first symptoms appear, ranges from a few days to three weeks. However, careful attention to wound hygiene will eliminate the possibility of tetanus in most cases. Deep puncture wounds and wounds with a lot of dead tissue should be thoroughly cleaned and not allowed to close until healing has occurred beneath the skin.[1]

Is tetanus a common and dangerous disease?

During the mid-1800s, there were 205 cases of tetanus per 100,000 wounds among U.S. military personnel. By the early 1900s, long before a tetanus vaccine was introduced, this rate had declined to 16 cases per 100,000 wounds—a 92 percent reduction. During the mid-1940s, tetanus dropped even further to .44 cases per 100,000 wounds.[2] Some researchers attribute this decline to an increased attention to wound hygiene.

Today, authorities claim that tetanus infects about 500,000 people each year worldwide, primarily in developing countries. However, many of these cases occur after a mother gives birth and the umbilical cord is cut with a dirty knife allowing tetanus spores to infect the newborn baby.[3] In the United States, from 1995 to 2005 (an 11-year period), there were just 386 total cases of tetanus—an average of 35 cases per year. Of this total, 43 people died—about four persons per year.[4] In Canada, there have been about four cases of tetanus annually in recent years, with no deaths recorded since 1997.[5]

The tetanus vaccine:

A tetanus vaccine became available in the 1920s. During the 1940s it was combined with diphtheria and pertussis vaccines. This became known as DPT. Today, the tetanus vaccine is most commonly administered in combination with both diphtheria and acellular pertussis vaccines (DTaP).

Daptacel, Infanrix, and Tripedia are the most common brands of DTaP, and how most children receive the tetanus vaccine. However, the tetanus vaccine is available without the pertussis component:

- DT (Diphtheria and Tetanus Toxoids Adsorbed)—A combination vaccine containing *Corynebacterium diphtheriae* cultures (diphtheria) and *Clostridium tetani* (tetanus) cultures made in a broth containing "bovine extract." Also contains sodium chloride, formaldehyde, 170mcg of aluminum, and "a trace amount of thimerosal." Multi-dose vials contain 25mcg of mercury per dose. Produced by Sanofi Pasteur. Indicated for children under 7 years of age. Given in 4 doses.[6]
- Decavac (Td)—A combination vaccine containing diphtheria and tetanus cultures grown in "an extract of bovine muscle tissue." Also contains sodium chloride, formaldehyde, 280mcg of aluminum, and "a trace amount of thimerosal." Produced by Sanofi Pasteur. Indicated for persons 7 years of age and older. Given in 3 doses.[7]

The tetanus vaccine can also be given by itself, without diphtheria or pertussis:

- TTa (Tetanus Toxoid Adsorbed)—*Clostridium tetani* (tetanus) culture "detoxified with formaldehyde." Also contains sodium chloride, sodium phosphate, 250mcg of aluminum and 25mcg of thimerosal. Produced by Sanofi Pasteur. Indicated for primary vaccination of persons 7 years of age and older. Given in 3 doses.[8]
- TT (Tetanus Toxoid Booster)—*Clostridium tetani* (tetanus) culture "detoxified with formaldehyde." Also contains sodium chloride and 25mcg of thimerosal. Does not contain aluminum. Produced by Sanofi Pasteur. Indicated for a booster injection—not primary vaccination—of persons 7 years of age and older.[9]

Several other combination vaccines with tetanus are available, including: Adacel (DTaP), Boostrix (DTaP), Kinrix (DTaP/Polio), TriHibit (DTaP/Hib), Pentacel (DTaP/Polio/Hib), and Pediarix (DTaP/Polio/Hep B).

Safety

Numerous studies and case reports have linked the tetanus vaccine to *severe* and even *fatal* side effects, including neurological and paralytic disorders such as Guillain-Barré syndrome (GBS), demyelinating diseases, immune disorders, arthritis, joint inflammation, asthma, allergies, anaphylactic shock, and other life-threatening reactions.[11]

A Tetanus Anti-Toxin is Available

A *tetanus immune globulin* (TIG) injection—an antitoxin—is also available. This shot may be given to persons with low tetanus antibody levels—*including unvaccinated individuals*—shortly after a serious wound occurs or if tetanus symptoms appear. This injection introduces tetanus-fighting antibodies directly into the body. The antibody levels achieved with TIG are often adequate to defend against the disease until your body can produce its own antibodies against tetanus.[12]

The tetanus vaccine and NEUROLOGICAL DISORDERS:

Tetanus vaccine manufacturers acknowledge in their own product inserts that neurological disorders such as Guillain-Barré syndrome (paralysis), brachial plexus neuropathies, and EEG disturbances with encephalopathy, have been reported following the shot.[13] In addition, "cases of demyelinating diseases of the central nervous system have been reported following some tetanus toxoid-containing vaccines or tetanus and diphtheria toxoid-containing vaccines."[14]

As early as 1966 the *Journal of the American Medical Association* documented peripheral neuropathy—damage to the central nervous system (CNS)—following the tetanus vaccine.[15] A few years later, *Archives of Neurology* described brachial plexus neuropathy—nerve damage and muscle weakness in the shoulders, arms and hands—after the tetanus shot.[16] Several other studies have documented neurological complications after the tetanus vaccine, including slurred speech, lethargy, a loss of sensation, transverse myelitis, and Guillain-Barré syndrome.[17-27] For example, *The Lancet* reported on an 11-year-old girl who developed optic neuritis and myelitis after she received a routine tetanus booster shot. She became blind from the vaccine, partially paralyzed in her legs, and lost control of her bladder.[28] Two years later, The U.S. Institute of Medicine (IOM) officially corroborated a causal relationship between the tetanus vaccine and brachial neuritis and Guillain-Barré syndrome.[29]

The tetanus vaccine and IMMUNE DISORDERS:

The *New England Journal of Medicine* published a study showing that tetanus booster vaccinations cause T-lymphocyte blood count ratios to drop below normal. The greatest decrease occurred up to two weeks later. The authors of the study noted that these altered ratios are similar to those found in victims of HIV/AIDS.[30] Even a brief suppression of normal T-lymphocyte ratios is undesirable, and may be the underlying cause of at least one immunological disorder found in infants.[31]

The tetanus vaccine and ARTHRITIS:

German scientists published a review of adverse reactions to the tetanus vaccine and documented several cases of "inflammatory changes of joints."[32] The *Annals of Rheumatic Disease* also found correlations between the tetanus vaccine and chronic joint inflammation. Laboratory tests were able to show that this vaccine can lead to rheumatoid arthritis.[33] In 1994, the U.S. Institute of Medicine chronicled several dozen cases of severe joint inflammation following the tetanus vaccine. When investigators conducted follow-up studies, it became evident that many of the victims had not recovered and were suffering long-term effects.[34]

Can the tetanus vaccine cause ASTHMA and ALLERGIES?

In 1997, *Epidemiology* published a study comparing asthma and allergy rates in unvaccinated children versus children who received a vaccine containing tetanus. None of the unvaccinated children had asthmatic episodes or health consultations for asthma or other allergic illnesses before 10 years of age. In the vaccinated children, 23 percent had asthmatic episodes and medical consultations for asthma, while 30 percent had medical consultations for other allergic illnesses. Similar differences were observed at 5 and 16 years of age.[35]

In 2000, a new study in the *Journal of Manipulative and Physiological Therapeutics* confirmed earlier findings that children who receive DPT or tetanus vaccines are significantly more likely to develop a "history of asthma" or other "allergy-related respiratory symptoms" than those who remain unvaccinated. The study included data from nearly 14,000 infants, children, and adolescents, aged 2 months to 16 years. A child who received the DPT or tetanus vaccine was 50 percent more likely to experience severe allergic reactions, 80 percent more likely to experience sinusitis, and twice as likely to develop asthma. In fact, the authors of the study calculated that "fifty percent of diagnosed asthma cases (2.93 million) in U.S. children and adolescents would be prevented if the DPT or tetanus shot was not administered. Similarly, 45 percent of sinusitis cases (4.94 million) and 54 percent of allergy-related episodes of nose and eye symptoms (10.54 million) in a 12-month period would be prevented after discontinuation of the vaccine."[36]

Anaphylaxis: The CDC reported that overly frequent injections of the tetanus vaccine may lead to allergic and hypersensitive reactions from very high antitoxin antibodies.[37,38] The tetanus vaccine manufacturer notes that "an anaphylactic reaction (hives, swelling of the mouth, difficulty breathing, hypotension, or shock) and death have been reported after receiving preparations containing tetanus and diphtheria antigens."[39] The Institute of Medicine also documented several cases of anaphylactic reactions—life-threatening allergic responses—within four hours of tetanus vaccines.[40] Earlier studies by German scientists already documented deaths resulting from anaphylactic reactions to the tetanus vaccine.[41,42]

VAERS: The case reports on the following page were taken directly from the FDA's Vaccine Adverse Event Reporting System (VAERS), a national database of suspected adverse reactions to mandatory shots.[43] They represent just a small sample of the potential harm associated with the tetanus vaccine. (Case numbers precede report summaries.) A personal case report resulting in death is included as well.[44]

Efficacy

Tetanus vaccine efficacy is usually determined by providing the shot to a small group of people and then measuring the number of tetanus-fighting antibodies produced in the blood. If this number meets or exceeds an officially established "protective level" then the vaccine is considered effective. For example, according to one manufacturer: "A clinical study to evaluate the serological responses...in 58 individuals...indicated protective levels were achieved in greater than 90 percent of the study population after primary immunization."[45] Another manufacturer states that: "A clinical study was performed in 20 children under one year of age to determine the serological responses.... Protective levels of...tetanus antitoxins were detected in 100 percent of the children following two doses of the vaccine."[46]

Again, if a predetermined number of antibodies are produced, the vaccine is considered effective. However, several studies and reports indicate that tetanus can occur in fully vaccinated people, that is, despite having tetanus antitoxin levels that are substantially above officially established protective levels.[47-49] For example, the *Canadian Medical Association Journal* recently documented a case of tetanus in a patient whose tetanus antitoxin titer "was more than 20 times higher than 'protective levels.'"[50]

Tetanus Vaccine: VAERS Case Reports

▶216727: A 4-month-old girl received the tetanus vaccine (DT) and 2 hours later developed a fever along with vomiting and diarrhea. The next morning, she had a seizure, and 3 more seizures at the hospital.

▶74630: A 10-month-old boy received the tetanus vaccine (DT) and 3 days later had a staring spell before falling back with all 4 limbs shaking. The baby became cyanotic with tremors lasting about 5 minutes.

▶99373: A 1-year-old girl received the tetanus vaccine (DT) and woke up the next morning unable to see.

▶298882: A 1-year-old boy received the tetanus vaccine (DT) in the morning and by early evening became "disoriented" and "would walk and then spontaneously fall down."

▶43425: A 1-year-old boy received the tetanus vaccine (DT) and three days later lost head control, his arms became weak, he developed labored breathing and subsequently died.

▶117249: A 2-year-old received the tetanus vaccine (T), developed a fever, became agitated and unable to move. Diagnosed with possible encephalitis.

▶288295: A 4-year-old female began "profusely bleeding from the nose" immediately after receiving the tetanus vaccine (DT).

▶166017: A 7-year-old boy received the tetanus vaccine (T), "developed complete paralysis from head to toes" and was hospitalized with GBS.

▶53533: A 10-year-old girl received the tetanus vaccine (T), collapsed and hit her head on the floor. Her pupils dilated and eyes rolled back, with "gaze palsy" and muscle twitching.

▶115055: An 11-year-old girl received the tetanus vaccine (T) and one day later lost strength in her legs, developed "visual deterioration" and lost control of her bowels and bladder. Symptoms included neuropathy, optic neuritis, myelitis, spastic paraparesis, and sensory loss.

Adverse Reactions in the Elderly

Young people are not the only groups susceptible to severe adverse reactions from the tetanus vaccine. Adults and the elderly make frequent reports as well. For example, one concerned woman wrote the following:

"My 78-year-old mother was given a tetanus shot in July in a hospital emergency room after a fall in her living room. She had scratched her nose with her eyeglasses, and they apparently give the shot routinely to anyone admitted with a scratch or cut. Within three hours, she was intubated, as her throat had closed and her tongue had swelled outside of her mouth. She also had some facial swelling. The ventilator was removed after four days. However, she wasn't able to swallow, eat, or breathe properly after that, and passed away seven days later."

Efficacy in the elderly: The geriatric population is especially susceptible to inadequate protection despite up-to-date vaccinations. However, the *Journal of the American Medical Association* published a study showing that vitamin E supplements boost immunity in elderly persons. Healthy elderly subjects who received a tetanus vaccine after ingesting 200 milligrams of vitamin E daily for more than 6 months produced more tetanus-fighting antibodies when compared to a similar group of elderly subjects who did not receive the vitamin E supplements.[51]

How many shots are necessary?

Authorities recommend five doses of the tetanus vaccine before a child enters school (usually administered via DTaP). A booster dose is expected at 11 to 12 years of age and every 10 years thereafter. According to one manufacturer, the tetanus vaccine "is a highly effective antigen... In a trial of 26 adults given a booster dose of tetanus toxoid, 81 percent demonstrated a 2-fold or greater rise in serum antitoxin antibody levels."[52] However, according to the eminent pediatrician Dr. Robert Mendelsohn...

"There is no credible scientific evidence indicating how often tetanus boosters are required. During the 1970s and 1980s, 40 percent of the child population was not protected yet tetanus infection rates continued to decline."[53]
—Robert Mendelsohn, MD, pediatrician

Should pregnant women get a tetanus vaccine?

The tetanus vaccine manufacturer warns pregnant women that "animal reproductive studies have not been conducted." Furthermore, "it is also not known whether [this vaccine] can cause fetal harm when administered to a pregnant woman or can affect reproductive capacity."[54] One mother describes her experience after receiving a tetanus vaccine during pregnancy:

"When I was three months pregnant I cut myself and was 'required' to get a tetanus shot. My son has been diagnosed with cerebral palsy and attention deficit disorder. He also has grand mal seizures, an enlarged liver and heart, and made no growth hormone at birth."[55]
—Mother who received a tetanus shot during pregnancy

Nursing mothers are warned as well: "It is not known whether [the tetanus vaccine] is excreted in human milk. Because many drugs are excreted in human milk, caution should be exercised when [the tetanus vaccine] is administered to a nursing woman."[56]

Notes

1. Skudder, PA., et al. "Current status of tetanus control: importance of human tetanus-immune globulin." *J of the American Medical Assoc.* 1964;188: 625-627.

2. Mortimer, E. "Immunization against infectious disease." *Science* (May 26, 1978); Volume 200:905.

3. World Health Organization. "Tetanus, the disease." www.who.int

4. CDC. Figures extracted from several *Morbidity and Mortality Weekly Reports (MMWR).*

5. Public Health Agency of Canada. "Vaccine-preventable diseases: tetanus." www.publichealth.gc.ca

6. Sanofi Pasteur. "DT—Diphtheria and Tetanus Toxoids Adsorbed USP (For Pediatric Use)." December 2005.

7. Sanofi Pasteur. "Decavac (Td)—Tetanus and Diphtheria Toxoids Adsorbed." December 2008.

8. Aventis Pasteur. "Tetanus Toxoid Adsorbed USP." April 1999.

9. Sanofi Pasteur. "Tetanus Toxoid (For Booster Use Only). December 2005.

11. See Notes 15-42

12. TalecrisBiotherapeutics. "HyperTET S/D." Product insert (2008).

13. See Notes 8 and 9.

14. Sanofi Pasteur. "Tripedia (Diphtheria and Tetanus Toxoids and Acellular Pertussis Vaccine Adsorbed.)" December 2005.

15. Blumstein, GI., et al. "Peripheral neuropathy following tetanus toxoid administration." *Journal of the American Medical Assoc* 1966;198:1030-1031.

16. Tsairis, P., et al. "Natural history of brachial plexus neuropathy." *Archives of Neurology* 1972;27:109-117.

17. Schlenska, GK. "Unusual neurological complications following tetanus toxoid administration." *Journal of Neurology* 1977;215:299-302.

18. Pollard, JD., et al. "Relapsing neuropathy due to tetanus toxoid." *Journal of the Neurological Sciences* 1978; 37:113-125.

19. Quast, U., et al. "Mono- and polyneuritis after tetanus vaccination." *Devel Bio Stand* 1979;43:25-32.

20. Reinstein, L., et al. "Peripheral neuropathy after multiple tetanus toxoid injections." *Archives Phys Med Rehabilitation* 1982;63:332-334.

21. Fenichel, GM. "Neurological complications of tetanus toxoid." *Archives of Neurology* 1983;40:390.

22. Holliday, PL., et al. "Polyradiculoneuritis secondary to immunization with tetanus and diphtheria toxoids." *Archives of Neurology* 1983;40:390.

23. Rutledge, SL., et al. "Neurologic complications of immunizations. *Journal of Pediatrics* 1986;109:917-924.

24. CDC. "Adverse events following immunization." *MMWR* 1985;34(3):43-47.

25. Newton, N., et al. "Guillain-Barré syndrome after vaccination with purified tetanus toxoid." *S Med J* 1987;80:1053-1054.

26. Schwartz, G., et al. "Acute midbrain syndrome as an adverse reaction to tetanus immunization." *Intensive Care Medicine* 1988;15:53-54.

27. Read, SJ., et al. "Acute transverse myelitis after tetanus toxoid vaccination." *The Lancet* 1992;339:1111-1112.

28. Topaloglu, H., et al. "Optic neuritis and myelitis after booster tetanus toxoid vaccination." *The Lancet* 1992; 339:178-179.

29. Institute of Medicine. *Adverse Events Associated with Childhood Vaccines: Evidence Bearing on Causality.* (Wash., DC: National Academy Press, 1994).

30. Eibl, M., et al. "Abnormal T-lymphocyte subpopulations in healthy subjects after

tetanus booster immunizations," *New England Journal of Medicine* (November 26, 1981): 1307-1313.

31. Buttram, H., et al. "Bringing vaccines into perspective," *Mothering Magazine* (Winter 1985):30.

32. Kroger, G., et al. "Tetanusimpfung: Vertraglichkeit und Vermeidung von Nebenreaktionen." [Tetanus vaccination: tolerance and avoidance of adverse reactions.] *Klininische Wochenschrift* 1986;64:767-775.

33. Jawad, AS., et al. "Immunisation triggering rheumatoid arthritis?" *Annals of Rheumatic Disease* 1989; 48:174.

34. See Note 29.

35. Kemp, T., et al. "Is infant immunization a risk factor for childhood asthma or allergy?" *Epidemiology* 1997;8(6):678-680.

36. Hurwitz, EL., et al. "Effects of diphtheria-tetanus-pertussis or tetanus vaccination on allergies and allergy-related respiratory symptoms among children and adolescents in the United States." *J of Manipulative & Physiological Therapeutics* 2000;23:1-10.

37. CDC. "Recommendations of the immunization practices advisory committee (ACIP): diphtheria, tetanus and pertussis: guidelines for vaccine prophylaxis and other preventive measures." *MMWR* 1985;34:405-426.

38. CDC. "Update: vaccine side effects, adverse reactions, contraindications, and precautions." *MMWR* 1996;45:22-31.

39. See Notes 6 and 8.

40. See Note 2.

41. Regamey, RH. Die Tetanus-Schutzimpfung. [Tetanus immunization in *Handbook of Immunization.*] In: Herrlick, A., ed. *Handbuch Schutzimpfungen* (Berlin: Springer, 1965).

42. Staak, M., et al. Zur problematik anaphylaktischer Reaktionen nach aktiver Tetanus-Immunisierung. [Anaphylactic reaction following active tetanus immunization.] *Deutsche Medizinische Wochenschrift* 1973; 98:110-111.

43. National Vaccine Information Center. "MedAlerts: access to the U.S. government's Vaccine Adverse Event Reporting System (VAERS)." www.medalerts.org

44. Thinktwice Global Vaccine Institute. Case report. www.thinktwice.com

45. See Note 7.

46. See Note 6.

47. Berger, SA., et al. "Tetanus despite preexisting anti-tetanus antibody." *Journal of the American Medical Association* 1978;240;769-770.

48. Passen, EL., et al. "Clinical tetanus despite a 'protective' level of toxin-neutralizing antibody." *Journal of the American Medical Association* 1986; 255:1171-1172.

49. Vieira, BI., et al. "Cephalic tetanus in an immunized patient." *Medical Journal of Australia* 1986;145:156-157.

50. Katz, KC., et al. "Postoperative tetanus: a case report." *Canadian Medical Association Journal* 2000; 163(5):571-573.

51. Meydani, SN., et al. "Vitamin E supplementation and in vivo immune response in healthy elderly subjects. A randomized controlled trial." *Journal of the American Medical Association* 1997;277(17): 1398-1399.

52. See Note 9.

53. Mendelsohn, R. *But Doctor, About That Shot...The Risks of Immunizations and How to Avoid Them.* (Evanston, IL: The People's Doctor Newsletter, 1988):4.

54. See Note 7.

55. See Note 44.

56. See Note 7.

Diphtheria

What is diphtheria

Diphtheria is a contagious bacterial disease of the upper respiratory system. It is mainly spread by the coughing and sneezing of infected persons. The first symptoms appear two to five days after infection. They include a sore throat, headache, coughing, fever, and swollen lymph nodes in the neck. As the disease progresses, a thick membrane forms on the surface of the tonsils and throat, and may extend into the windpipe and lungs. This membrane may interfere with breathing and swallowing. In severe cases, it can completely block the breathing passages and cause death if not treated. Other complications include inflammation of the heart muscle and respiratory paralysis.

Diphtheria requires medical attention but is treatable with common antibiotics such as penicillin. Heart failure is treated with medication, while a respirator is used to aid in breathing. A diphtheria antitoxin may also be administered.

Is diphtheria a common disease?

Diphtheria was a common disease during the late 19th century. The case-fatality rate was about five percent. In the United States during the 1940s, the number of diphtheria cases fluctuated between 15,000 and 30,000 annually.[1] However, in 1980 a new pattern emerged, with only a few cases occurring each year. From 1995 to 2005 (an 11-year period), there were just 14 cases of diphtheria—about one case per year. Four of these cases were fatal.[2]

The diphtheria vaccine:

A diphtheria antitoxin became available in 1895 and was used on a limited scale from the start of the 20th century through the early 1940s. It supplied the body with a quick infusion of antibodies. It was given to people with low diphtheria antibody levels or shortly after being exposed to the disease. Today, a diphtheria antitoxin is still available. It is made from the blood of horses after they are inoculated with diphtheria organisms.

A diphtheria vaccine was introduced in the 1920s. However, widespread use did not occur until the 1940s when it was combined with the tetanus and pertussis vaccines. This became known as DPT. Today, the diphtheria toxoid is administered in conjunction with the tetanus vaccine (DT), or in combination with both tetanus and acellular pertussis vaccines (DTaP).

Safety

In 1924, the *Journal of the American Medical Association* cited several cases of suffering and death following diphtheria antitoxin:

- Case #1: Antitoxin was given, and immediately the patient felt a lump in her stomach. Five minutes later she had tingling, restlessness, followed by convulsions, cyanosis and respiratory failure. Three minutes later her heart stopped. Death occurred in eight minutes.
- Case #2: Seven minutes after antitoxin injection, the patient had itching on the body and scalp, then suddenly broke out with large "confluent wheals." There was nausea and vomiting. A severe convulsion was followed by death 35 minutes from time of injection.
- Case #3: A strong healthy child received diphtheria inoculation, had a sudden reaction and died in five minutes.
- Case #4: A school boy was given a prophylactic injection of antitoxin; he reacted and died in 20 minutes.
- Case #5: Five minutes after injection, the patient became apprehensive. The heartbeat continued 15 minutes after respiration ceased; death occurred 20 minutes after injection.
- Case #6: The patient was given antitoxin. Two minutes later, it had gone to his stomach. He began to choke, became cyanotic and collapsed. Death occurred in five minutes.
- Case #7: The patient was given a prophylactic dose of serum, collapsed and fell from his chair. Death occurred in ten minutes.[3]

In 1929, the *Journal of the American Medical Association* conducted a survey in which physicians were asked about the diphtheria vaccine and antitoxin therapy. More than 1,200 doctors participated. Over 90 percent of them stated that they oppose diphtheria inoculations:

> *"[We] do not favor or use [diphtheria antitoxin therapy] or consider the injection of diphtheria vaccine a satisfactory method of treatment. The reactions were too severe and the deaths and permanent disability were too frequent to justify its use."[4]*
> **—Quote from doctors, published in *JAMA***

In 1938, *The Lancet* astounded the scientific community when it published a blunt admission by a respected medical doctor of diphtheria vaccine safety problems:

"Suppose we include in our propaganda a candid account of the various untoward 'accidents' which have accompanied [diphtheria vaccination]. If we badly told the whole truth it is doubtful whether the public would submit to inoculation."[5]
—**Dr. D.C. Okell**

Today, the diphtheria toxoid is administered in conjunction with the tetanus vaccine (DT), or in combination with both tetanus and acellular pertussis vaccines (DTaP). Thus, adverse reactions are difficult to attribute to any single component of the shot. For more information about the potential side effects of this vaccine, read the chapters on tetanus and pertussis (including DTaP).

Efficacy

The diphtheria death rate continued to plummet long before the vaccine was introduced. In the United States, from 1900 to 1930, diphtheria fatalities declined by more than 85 percent.[6] In fact, mortality from the disease decreased from 7.2 deaths per 10,000 in 1911 to 0.9 deaths per 10,000 in 1935—an 88 percent decline.[7]

In 1969, there was an outbreak of diphtheria in Chicago, Illinois. The city Board of Health reported that 38 percent of the cases had been fully vaccinated or showed serological evidence of full immunity. More than 50 percent of the cases had been partially or completely vaccinated prior to contracting the disease.[8] A report on another outbreak revealed that 14 of 23 infected persons (61 percent) had been fully vaccinated.[9]

In 1975, the Food and Drug Administration confessed that diphtheria may occur in vaccinated individuals:

"[The diphtheria vaccine] is not as effective an immunizing agent as might be anticipated... The permanence of immunity induced by the toxoid...is open to question."[10]
—**FDA**

In 1979, authorities changed the medical definition of diphtheria. Prior to the change, "skin" and "inhalation" cases of the disease were counted. After the change, only inhalation cases were labeled as bona fide diphtheria. As a result, official statistics showed an immediate 95 percent drop in cases the following year (and a 99.3 percent drop from 1970 to 1980). The number of cases remained low every year thereafter.[11,12]

Notes

1. CDC. Data published in several *Morbidity and Mortality Weekly Reports.*

2. CDC. "Reported cases and deaths from vaccine preventable diseases, US, 1950-2005." *Pink Book,* (Dec 13, 2006).

3. *Journal of the American Medical Association* (April 15, 1924).

4. *Journal of the American Medical Association* (March 16, 1929).

5. *The Lancet* (January 1938).

6. Alderson, M. *International Mortality Statistics* (Washington, DC: Facts on File, 1981).

7. Dublin, L., et al. *Twenty-Five Years of Health Progress* (New York: Metro-politan Life Insurance Company, 1937):60.

8. Mendelsohn, R. *How to Raise a Healthy Child...In Spite of Your Doctor.* (Ballantine Books, 1984):245.

9. Ibid.

10. FDA. "Minutes of the 15th meeting of the panel of review of bacterial vaccines and toxoids with standards and potency." *Bureau of Biologics* (November 20-21, 1975).

11. CDC. "Summary of notifiable diseases, 1999." *MMWR* (April 6, 2001);48(53):84-90.

12. Physician's Desk Reference (PDR); 55th edition. (Montvale, NJ: Medical Economics, 2001):787.

Pertussis
(DPT and DTaP)

What is pertussis?

Pertussis is a contagious disease caused by a bacterium that affects the respiratory system. Sometimes called whooping cough, this disease got its name from the high-pitched whooping noise victims make when they try to catch their breath after severe coughing attacks. Symptoms progress through three stages. In the first stage, which usually lasts one to two weeks, victims have trouble breathing, and may develop a cough and fever. In the second stage, which usually lasts two to three weeks, severe coughing attacks occur during the night, and then later during the day and night. The attacks can lead to inadequate oxygen, which can cause convulsions. During this stage death can occur. In the final stage, coughing lessens and recovery begins. Full recovery may take two to three months.

How prevalent and serious is pertussis?

Pertussis epidemics were relatively common in Europe during the 16th, 17th and 18th centuries. Outbreaks were also common in America. By the 1930s, 73 percent of all U.S. children under 10 were exposed to the disease and a small percentage died.[1] Today, pertussis is rarely fatal.[2] However, when infants under six months contract the disease, it can be serious and life-threatening. There is no specific treatment for pertussis. Antibiotics and cough suppressants have been used, but with little effect, and are generally not recommended.

The pertussis vaccine:

The first "whole-cell" pertussis vaccine was developed in the early 1900s and put into general use during the mid-1930s and early 1940s. In 1946, the pertussis vaccine was mixed with vaccines for diphtheria and tetanus. This became known as DPT, the world's first "three-in-one" combination shot. In 1981, Japan replaced DPT with DTaP because it contains a supposedly safer "acellular" form of pertussis. The United States switched from DPT to DTaP in 1996.

The CDC and vaccine manufacturers recommend 5 doses of DTaP for infants and children prior to 7 years of age. (Read the Recommended Immunization Schedule, endorsed by the CDC and American Academy of Pediatrics, for more information.) Today, DTaP is available in three different brands:

- Daptacel—Contains 330mcg of aluminum, formaldehyde, 2-phenoxyethanol and glutaraldehyde. Produced by Sanofi Pasteur.
- Infanrix—Contains 625mcg of aluminum, formaldehyde, bovine casein, polysorbate 80, and glutaraldehyde. Produced by GSK.
- Tripedia—Contains 170mcg of aluminum, formaldehyde, gelatin, bovine extract, polysorbate 80, sodium chloride, sodium phosphate, and "a trace amount of thimerosal." Produced by Sanofi Pasteur.

Some brands of DTaP include the polio, Hib and hepatitis B vaccines as well—"4-in-one" and "5-in-one" combination shots:
- Pentacel—A combination vaccine for DTaP, inactivated polio, and Hib. Contains 330mcg of aluminum, formaldehyde, polysorbate 80, glutaraldehyde, 2-phenoxyethanol, calf serum, neomycin, and polymyxin B sulfate. Polio viruses are grown in MRC-5 human diploid cells (cultured from aborted human fetuses). Produced by Sanofi Pasteur. Given in 4 doses.
- Pediarix—A combination vaccine for DTaP, inactivated polio, and hepatitis B. Contains 850mcg of aluminum, formaldehyde, polysorbate 80, glutaraldehyde, bovine extract, neomycin sulfate, polymyxin B, sodium chloride, and yeast protein. Polio viruses are grown in Vero cells (from monkey kidneys). Produced by GSK. Given in 3 doses.
- TriHIBit—A combination vaccine for DTaP and Hib. (This shot combines Tripedia with ActHIB.) Used as a booster dose only.
- Kinrix—A combination vaccine for DTaP and inactivated polio. (This shot contains the same DTaP and polio components found in Pediarix.) Used as a booster dose only.[3]

Two different brands of Tdap—similar to DTaP, except with less diphtheria and pertussis—are available for teens and adults: Adacel and Boostrix. They are for booster doses only.

Safety

The pertussis vaccine has been linked to high fever, pain, diarrhea, projectile vomiting, persistent crying, high-pitched screaming, (the cri encephalique, or encephalitic scream associated with central nervous system damage), brain disorders, seizures, convulsions, physical disabilities, learning disorders, anaphylactic reactions, collapse, shock, respiratory problems, asthma, autism, and sudden infant death syndrome (SIDS).[4]

The pertussis vaccine and NEUROLOGICAL DISORDERS:

The DPT vaccine has a long, well-documented history of causing severe, irreversible and fatal reactions in previously healthy children. For example, as early as 1933, the *Journal of the American Medical Association* published data showing dangerous side effects—cyanosis and convulsions—after pertussis vaccinations.[5] In 1948, *Pediatrics* published details of several children who had persistent neurological damage, including coma, cerebral palsy, mental retardation, and death, after their pertussis vaccinations.[6]

In the 1950s, *The Lancet,* the *Journal of Pediatrics,* and the *British Medical Journal* all published reports documenting more than 100 cases of infantile myoclonic seizures, mental retardation and paralysis in children after their DPT shots.[7-10] In 1974, the Royal Society of Medicine held a conference in which authorities questioned whether the pertussis vaccine "outweighs the damage which it may be doing."[11] In 1977, a Scottish study analyzed 160 cases of DPT reactions, many of which were "followed by convulsions, hyperkinesis [attention deficit hyperactivity disorder] and severe mental defect." The author of the study concluded that "most adverse reactions are unreported and...overlooked."[12]

In 1981, the *British Medical Journal* investigated nearly 1,200 children who were hospitalized with neurological illness. Researchers concluded that DPT vaccination had occurred significantly more often within 72 hours, and within 7 days, prior to the damage, than in control subjects who did not exhibit neurological impairment.[13] In 1993, authors of a study published in the *British Medical Journal* concluded that the pertussis-vaccinated children "were significantly more likely than controls to have died or to have some form of educational, behavioral, neurological, or physical dysfunction" ten years after their initial adverse reaction.[14]

The pertussis vaccine and ASTHMA:

In 1994, the *Journal of the American Medical Association* published data showing that children diagnosed with asthma were five times more likely than not to have received the pertussis vaccine.[15] In 1997, *Epidemiology* published a study comparing children who had been vaccinated with pertussis to children who did not receive the pertussis vaccine. More than 20 percent of the pertussis-vaccinated children developed asthma within 5 to 10 years, whereas none of the children in the control group acquired the ailment.[16] In 1998, a study published in *Thorax* showed a 1.4-fold increased risk of asthma associated with pertussis vaccination.[17] In 2000, a new study showed that children who received DPT or tetanus vaccines were significantly more likely to develop a "history of asthma" or other "allergy-related respiratory symptoms" than those who remained unvaccinated.[18] In 2008, the *Journal of Allergy and Clinical Immunology* published a study of 11,531 children who received DPT and found that babies vaccinated on schedule were twice as likely to develop asthma when compared to babies whose first DPT shots were delayed.[19] That same year, *Pediatric Allergy and Immunology* published a study showing that pertussis-vaccinated babies were more than twice as likely to develop atopic disorders—asthma, hay fever and food allergies—by 8-12 years of age, when compared to unvaccinated children.[20]

The pertussis vaccine and AUTISM:

The first cases of autism in the United States occurred at a time shortly after the pertussis vaccine became available in the 1930s and 1940s. During the 1960s, mass vaccination campaigns were instituted. The growing number of children suffering from this new illness directly coincided with the increasing popularity of the mandated immunization programs during these same years. Europe began promoting the pertussis vaccine in the 1950s; the first cases of autism began to appear on that continent in the same decade. In England, the pertussis vaccine wasn't promoted on a large scale until the late 1950s. Shortly thereafter, the first autism support organization in the United Kingdom was required and established.[21]

The pertussis vaccine and DEVELOPMENTAL DISABILITIES:

According to the medical historian, Harris L. Coulter, Ph.D., the entire post World War II generation is suffering from "post-encephalitic syndrome" —the name he gives to define a variety of vaccine-induced disabilities.[22] Coulter presented evidence showing that the long-term effects of pertussis shots may be more pervasive than suspected. However, injuries caused by the pertussis vaccine are often "disguised" under different names: autism, dyslexia, learning disability, epilepsy, hyperactivity (ADHD), delinquency, antisocial behavior, and mental retardation, to name a few.[23] The developmental disabilities and other conditions noted above may be caused by encephalitis, or inflammation of the brain. Medical practitioners know that encephalitis can be caused by a severe injury to the head, from an infectious disease, *or from the vaccines against these diseases* —post-vaccinal encephalitis.[24] According to Dr. Coulter:

"The principal cause of encephalitis in the United States today, and in other industrialized countries as well, is childhood vaccination programs."[25]
—**Dr. Harris Coulter, medical historian**

The symptoms of post-vaccinal encephalitis are identical to the symptoms of encephalitis arising from any other cause. Since any segment of the nervous system may be affected, every possible physical, intellectual, and personality deviation, and combinations of them, are possible.[26-28] Autopsies after post-vaccinal encephalitis show a loss and destruction of myelin on the brainstem and spinal cord. Myelin covers and protects the nerves much like the insulation on an electric wire. Without myelin, nerve impulses are short-circuited and the nervous system remains undeveloped and immature.[29] An overt reaction to the pertussis vaccine is not required to confirm that post-vaccinal encephalitis, or damage to the central nervous system, occurred. In fact, there is no correlation between the degree of cerebral damage that may later ensue and the severity of the reaction that led to encephalitis in the first place. In other words, subtle and often overlooked reactions to the vaccine (i.e., a fever, fussiness, drowsiness) can be, and often is, a case of encephalitis which is capable of causing severe neurological complications months or even years later.[30-34]

Antisocial behavior: A disproportionate amount of antisocial behavior is committed by people with neurological damage. As early as the 1920s researchers were aware that children who had "recovered" from encephalitis were more likely to engage in misconduct and harmful behavior. They were called "apaches."[35-37] Today we call these children juvenile delinquents, often suffering from attention deficit or conduct disorder, but their numbers are now epidemic and their crimes more violent. Studies confirm that children with neurologically based disorders often engage in violent criminal behavior as adolescents and adults.[38] In one study, hyperactive children were twenty times more likely than the rest of the population to end up in a reform school.[39] A report in the *Journal of the American Medical Association* acknowledged that a disproportionate number of felons suffered from hyperactivity disorder (ADHD) during their earlier years.[40]

Perceptive parents may notice the onset of antisocial behavior in their children after their shots. One mother describes her experience:

"After my child received his shots at six months, he had high fever, screaming, and convulsions. The doctor said these reactions are normal side effects. From that day on my easygoing, happy, baby boy became what he is today. The last five years have been filled with life revolving around his moods. He goes from happy to outraged in seconds, has impulsive fits and hurts his siblings, argues with everything and everyone, can't focus or sit still. It was so confusing and scary to see this all start in a six-month-old baby."[41]

Another mother describes her experience:

"My son was born perfectly healthy. He had a bad reaction after his first vaccines—inconsolable crying for 12 hours. The doctor told me to never give him another pertussis shot. And we didn't. As time went by we noticed that he didn't learn from discipline. Then, as he got older he couldn't tell the truth even if he wanted something that he was offered. We struggled, reached out for help, took him to a psychiatrist. He has no impulse control; he knows right from wrong but when put in a situation, he can't choose right if his life depended on it. I have believed for many years that this vaccine caused brain damage, but I can't get anyone to order a brain scan. He is almost 17 and is going to juvenile prison for the second time. Who is tracking these kids? How do we know that these vaccines aren't causing bipolar, antisocial disorder, mood disorders or ADHD? Certainly vaccines are what these children have in common. If a child has a seizure or dies after a vaccine, that is reported, but who is watching out for all these kids who have had 'milder' reactions?"[42]

The pertussis vaccine and Sudden Infant Death Syndrome (SIDS):
In the 1960s and 1970s, Aborigine infants began to mysteriously die at astonishing rates. In some regions of Australia, 1 of every 2 babies succumbed to an unexplained death—a fatality rate of 50 percent! Dr. Archie Kalokerinos solved the riddle when he realized the deaths were occurring after the babies were vaccinated against pertussis and other diseases. Health officials had recently initiated a mass vaccination campaign to "protect" Aborigine babies; their deaths corresponded with the program. Evidently, these babies were severely malnourished, especially deficient in vitamin C. When they were vaccinated, their undeveloped immune systems couldn't handle the additional stress. Dr. Kalokerinos was able to save other babies from the same fate by administering small quantities of vitamin C (100mg per month of age) prior to their shots.[43]
In Japan, from 1970 to 1974, there were 37 documented infant deaths following pertussis vaccinations.[44] Doctors boycotted the vaccine, and in 1975 Japanese authorities raised the age of vaccination from two months to two years. As a result, babies stopped dying unexpectedly. In fact, the Japanese infant mortality rate improved from 17th place to best in the world.[45] According to scientists writing in *Pediatrics*...

"The category of 'sudden death' is instructive in that the entity disappeared following both whole-cell and acellular vaccines when immunization was delayed until a child was 24 months of age."[46]
—Observation made by scientists in *Pediatrics*

In 1987, the *American Journal of Public Health* published a study that found "the SIDS mortality rate in the period zero to three days following DPT to be 7.3 times that in the period beginning 30 days after immunization."[47] A 1992 study reported that babies die at a rate *8 times* greater than normal within 3 days after getting a DPT shot.[48] A remarkable Australian study of SIDS (cot death) measured episodes of apnea (cessation of breathing) and hypopnea (abnormally shallow breathing) before and after pertussis shots. A sophisticated microprocessor was placed under each baby's mattress to measure precise breathing patterns. The data clearly revealed that pertussis vaccination caused an excessive increase in episodes where breathing either nearly ceased or stopped completely. Dr. Viera Scheibner, the main author of the study, concluded that "vaccination is the single most prevalent and most preventable cause of infant deaths."[49-52]

In another study of children who died of SIDS, Dr. William Torch found that two-thirds had been vaccinated with pertussis prior to death. Dr. Torch also found that unvaccinated babies who died of SIDS did so most often in the fall or winter while vaccinated babies died most often at 2 and 4 months—the same ages when initial doses of pertussis are given to infants. Dr. Torch concluded that...

> *"DPT may be a generally unrecognized major cause of sudden infant and early childhood death, and that the risks of immunization may outweigh its potential benefits. A need for reevaluation and possible modification of current vaccination procedures is indicated by this study."*[53]
> **—Dr. William Torch, SIDS researcher**

The discontinued "whole-cell" DPT vaccine is not the only pertussis shot linked to SIDS. The current, supposedly safer "acellular" DTaP vaccine may cause infant deaths as well. One mother describes her experience:

> *"I had a child die of SIDS. I dug out his shot records and baby book only to find that he had the DTaP vaccine just three weeks prior to his death, and during those three weeks, my records show that I had him to the pediatrician four times for respiratory infection and two times to the emergency room for respiratory distress. These symptoms began within two days after the administration of the shot! I am convinced after my research that the DTaP is responsible for his death. The three precious children I have left will not receive another vaccine!"*[54]
> **—Mother of a child who died after receiving DTaP**

DTaP

In 1981, Japan began giving their children a new "acellular" pertussis vaccine (DTaP). They claimed it was less dangerous than the standard "whole-cell" vaccine (DPT) used in the United States. However, in 1975, a few years before the new pertussis vaccine was introduced in Japan, authorities raised the starting age of vaccination to two years. In the United States, pertussis shots are begun at two months, and are continued throughout the infant's early, high risk months. Thus it has been difficult to determine whether the acellular vaccine is truly safer.[55]

Is DTaP safer than DPT?

In 1987, the *Journal of the American Medical Association* reported that the DTaP vaccine reduced "mild" vaccine reactions by 60 percent when compared to the DPT shot. However, the new acellular DTaP vaccine and the original whole-cell DPT shot had similar rates of *severe* reactions.[56] That same year, 66 victims of the Japanese acellular pertussis vaccine won huge awards from their government. The court recognized that the authorities were denying adverse reactions so that the "public interest in preventing contagious diseases" wouldn't be undermined.[57]

In 1988, a Swedish study documented several deaths in babies who received the acellular vaccine. This led Swedish authorities to recommend withdrawing their application to license the shot.[58] In 1989, *Pediatrics* published the results of another Swedish study confirming fewer mild reactions with the DTaP vaccine, but children were still succumbing to unusual, prolonged crying—the cri encephalique—hypotonic reactions, and encephalitis. In fact, 1 of every 106 DTaP-vaccinated babies had serious adverse reactions such as inflammation of the brain—a much higher rate than official figures for the whole-cell DPT vaccine.[59]

In 1996, U.S. authorities replaced DPT with the DTaP vaccine for all five doses—despite concerns by some vaccine research organizations, including the National Vaccine Information Center, that...

"Most of the mild and serious reactions which have been reported following DPT vaccination have also been reported following DTaP."[60]
  —**National Vaccine Information Center**

What do the DTaP vaccine manufacturers say?

A recent check of the most current product data sheets published by DTaP vaccine manufacturers—as of July 2009—revealed dire warnings of irreversible risks and an extensive list of serious adverse reactions that have been reported following receipt of the DTaP shot. The following list includes "events which have a probable causal connection to components" of the DTaP vaccine: anaphylactic reactions, encephalopathy, neuropathy, brachial neuritis, Guillain-Barré syndrome, demyelinating diseases of the central nervous system, lymphadenopathy, bulging fontanelle, cranial mononeuropathy, seizures, grand mal convulsions, high-pitched cry, persistent cry, screaming, hypotonic/hyporesponsive episodes, cellulitis, cyanosis, thrombocytopenia, anorexia, diarrhea, vomiting, ear pain, autism, apnea, difficulty breathing, and sudden infant death syndrome (SIDS).[61]

Efficacy

The incidence and severity of whooping cough had begun to decline long before the pertussis vaccine was introduced. From 1900 to 1935, the death rate from pertussis in the United States had already declined on its own by 79 percent. In the United Kingdom, the death rate from pertussis had declined by 82 percent during this same period.[62]

A Swedish study evaluated two different acellular pertussis vaccines and concluded they were 54 and 64 percent effective, respectively.[63] As a result, Swedish officials asserted that "the efficacy of the [DTaP] vaccine may be lower than that of whole-cell vaccines."[64] On this basis, along with some concerns about safety issues, they withdrew their application to license the shot.[65] However, a German study claims greater efficacy —about 80 percent—but only after "adjusting" for sibling age, number of siblings in day care, well-baby visits, and father's employment status![66]

A 2006 Canadian study suggests that the current DTaP vaccine is not as effective as the older DPT shot, and may not protect young children.[67] A 2007 study published in *Clinical Infectious Diseases* found that five years after adolescents received an acellular pertussis booster shot (their 6th pertussis vaccine!) pertussis antibody levels were actually *lower* than they were before vaccination. In fact, they were *undetectable* in 28 percent of the subjects.[67]

Vaccine failures: In 1993, during a pertussis outbreak in Ohio, 82 percent of younger children stricken with the disease had received multiple doses of the vaccine.[68] That same year, during a large pertussis outbreak in Alberta, Canada, 62 percent of the people who contracted the disease had received their "age-appropriate" shots.[69]

DTaP Vaccine: VAERS Case Reports

The case reports below were taken directly from the FDA's Vaccine Adverse Event Reporting System (VAERS). They are just a small sample of the potential harm associated with DTaP.[70]

▸187791: A 3-month-old boy received DTaP and died 5 hours later.

▸122084: A 4-month-old girl received DTaP and 18 hours later had seizures. Four days later she had a sudden loss of consciousness, with apnea, hypotonia, hypoxia, cyanosis, unresponsive episodes in the hospital, gastrointestinal disorder, and a delay with walking.

▸253739: A 5-month-old girl received DTaP and died the following day. The autopsy states that the child was well on the day of vaccination, then developed fever, severe diarrhea, and vomited. She became limp, the care giver started CPR, and the child was transported to ER.

▸150475: A 6-month-old baby received DTaP "two days prior to arrival at ER in full cardiac arrest." The autopsy listed the cause of death as SIDS.

▸311936: A 6-month-old girl received her 3rd dose of DTaP, developed a fever and "hemorrhagic rash." She died the following day.

▸124771: One day after a 7-month-old girl received DTaP she was found unresponsive and could not be resuscitated.

▸98504: A 10-month-old boy received DTaP and two days later developed "pulmonal spasms" and a "barking cough" with asthma.

▸110709: A 10-month-old girl received DTaP and later that evening developed a high fever, an abnormal EEG, with staring episodes and convulsions. She also developed a "gait disturbance" and began to stumble.

▸133897: An 11-month-old boy received DTaP and was found "cold and limp" by his mother later that afternoon during his nap. The cause of death was listed as "acute pulmonary decompensation."

▸154929: A 15-month-old boy received DTaP and developed a fever, cough, runny nose and rash. Three days later he developed "edema of the extremities, hyperemic conjunctiva, and strawberry tongue." He was diagnosed with Kawasaki disease and hospitalized. He was also diagnosed with lymphadenopathy, Stevens-Johnson syndrome and "toxic epidermal necrolysis."

▸186491: A 2-year-old boy received DTaP and developed "abnormal behavior, aggression, cognitive disorder, neurodevelopmental disorder, obsessive-compulsive disorder, psychomotor hyperactivity, and sleep disorder." Also: persistent crying, screaming, decreased ability for eye contact and responses, hyperactivity, tantrums, loss of language and concentration, developmental delay, severe diarrhea, stomach pain, food allergies, and impaired socialization.

▸68561: A 2½-year-old girl received DTaP and later that evening she collapsed, went into cardiac arrest, and died.

DTaP Vaccine: Case Reports by Parents

▸ *"My son was given DTaP three days ago. Yesterday he had a temperature of 102 with no appetite. He has been jerking while he sleeps and has not been himself. The doctor said that because it was three days later it wasn't the shot. Now I am kicking myself for letting them convince me it was okay."*

▸ *"My son is one year old. On his 9-month visit, he received the DTaP shot. The next two days he was doing a strange sort of jerking movement with his face. It looked like a mini-seizure. His body would tighten up when they would occur. I am now worried about getting the next DTaP shot."*

▸ *"They gave my daughter DTaP after they told me there were no known side effects. They threatened to call Child Protection if I refused. The fear of losing her loomed over me, so I let her have it. Within minutes of arriving home she began to scream like I had never heard before. She screamed for 16 hours, with no break. The doctor swore that she was okay and just 'colicky.' After screaming, she became lethargic. She wouldn't even look up when I said her name. She had a seizure and went to the hospital. My daughter now receives only the DT shot, and although the nurses get angry, I insist to see the label of the shot bottle before any injections are given to her."* [71]

In 1996, there was a statewide outbreak of pertussis in Vermont, where 97 percent of all children 19-35 months of age were properly vaccinated. Yet, their pertussis shots were not effective because 74 percent of all children 7 months to 4 years of age who were stricken with the disease had received 3 to 5 doses of the vaccine. In addition, 68 percent of all 7-18 year-olds who caught pertussis had received 4 or 5 doses of the shot.[72]

In 2003, there was a large pertussis outbreak in Cyprus despite a pertussis vaccination rate of 98 percent. According to researchers, "most cases in the outbreak had previously been vaccinated for pertussis." In fact, 79 percent of everyone who contracted the disease had received 3 to 5 doses of the vaccine; just 13 percent were completely unvaccinated.[73]

In Israel, cases of pertussis rose 16-fold between 1998 and 2004, even though "national pertussis immunization coverage by age 2 years was stable during the last ten years."[74] (Nearly 93 percent of all 2-year-olds had received 4 doses of the pertussis vaccine.) In Israel, the acellular pertussis vaccine was introduced in 2002. From 2003 through 2005, compliance to pertussis vaccination actually *increased,* but pertussis incidence continued to climb.[75]

In 2009, there was a pertussis outbreak in New Jersey; *all* (100 percent) of the children who caught the disease were fully vaccinated against it.[77]

Pertussis in older age groups:
During the 1980s, 1990s and 2000s, the number of pertussis cases among adolescents and adults substantially *increased,* despite high vaccination rates. Before the pertussis vaccine was introduced, more than 93 percent of all cases occurred in children. However, the vaccine shifted the epidemiological patterns of the disease. Today, the majority of cases are in adolescents and adults.[76] Thus, authorities now recommend booster shots for people in these age groups.

Is the pertussis vaccine mandatory?
The CDC recommends 5 doses of DTaP for infants and children up to 7 years of age. However, a two month old baby weighing less than ten pounds receives the same dose of pertussis vaccine as a 50 pound child entering preschool. A DT shot (diphtheria and tetanus, without pertussis) is available for parents who are concerned about DTaP, although adverse reactions have been linked to the diphtheria and tetanus vaccines as well. Childhood vaccines are not legally required in most states.

Notes

1. Coulter, HL. and Fisher, BL. *A Shot in the Dark: Why the P in DPT Vaccination May be Hazardous to Your Child's Health* (Garden City Park, NY: Avery Pub Group, 1991):4-6.

2. CDC. "Summary of notifiable diseases, United States, 2003." *MMWR* (April 22, 2005);52 (54):78; Table 12: Deaths from selected notifiable diseases—United States, 1996-2001.

3. Product inserts by vaccine manufacturers: Daptacel (March 2008); Infanrix (2009); Tripedia (2005); Pentacel (June 2008); Pediarix (October 2008); ActHIB (December 2005); Kinrix (2009).

4. See Notes 5-21, 41, 43, 47-53, 56-60, and 70.

5. Madsen, T. "Vaccination against whooping cough." *JAMA* 1933;101(3):187-88.

6. Byers, RK., et al. "Encephalopathies following prophylactic pertussis vaccine." *Pediatrics* 1948;1(4):437-57.

7. Anderson, IM., et al. "Encephalopathy after combined diphtheria-pertussis inoculation." *The Lancet* (Mar 25, 1950):537-39.

8. Low, NL. "Electroencephalographic studies following pertussis immunizations." *Journal of Pediatrics* 1955;47:35-39.

9. Baird, HW., et al. "Infantile myoclonic seizures." *Journal of Pediatrics* 1957; 50:332-39.

10. Berg, JM. "Neurological complications of pertussis immunization." *British Medical Journal* (July 5, 1958):24-27.

11. Dick, G. "Convulsive disorders in young children." *Proceedings of the Royal Society of Medicine* 1974;67:371-72.

12. Stewart, GT. "Vaccination against whooping cough: efficacy vs. risks." *The Lancet* (January 29, 1977):234-37.

13. Miller, DL., et al. "Pertussis immunisation and serious neurological illness in children." *British Medical Journal* 1981;282:1595-99.

14. Miller, DL., et al. "Pertussis immunisation and serious acute neurological illnesses in children." *British Medical Journal* 1993;307:1171-76.

15. Odent, M., et al. "Pertussis vaccination and asthma: is there a link?" *Journal of the American Medical Association* (August 24/31, 1994):592-93.

16. Kemp, T., et al. "Is infant immunization a risk factor for childhood asthma or allergy?" *Epidemiology* 1997;8:678-80.

17. Farooqi, IS., et al. "Early childhood infection and atopic disorder." *Thorax* 1998;53:927-32.

18. Hurwitz, EL., et al. "Effects of diphtheria-tetanus-pertussis or tetanus vaccination on allergies and allergy-related respiratory symptoms among children and adolescents in the United States." *J of Manipulative and Physiological Therapeutics* 2000;23:1-10.

19. McDonald, KL., et al. "Delay in diphtheria, pertussis, tetanus vaccination is associated with a reduced risk of childhood asthma." *J Allergy Clin Immunology* 2008;121(3):626-31.

20. Bernsen, R., et al. "Reported pertussis infection and risk of atopy in 8- to 12-yr-old vaccinated and non-vaccinated children." *Pediatric Allergy and Immun* 2008;19(1):46-52.

21. Coulter, HL. *Vaccination, Social Violence, and Criminality: The Medical Assault on the American Brain* (Berkeley, CA: North Atlantic Books, 1990):50.

22. Leviton, R. "A Shot in the Dark," *Yoga Journal* (May/June, 1992):112-114.

23. See Note 21, pp. ix-xvi; Chapters 1-5.

24. See Note 21, pp. xiii-xiv; Chapters 1-5.

25. See Note 21, p. xiv.

26. See Note 21, p. 103.

27. Merritt, HH. *Textbook of Neurology,* 6th Ed. (Philadelphia, PA:Lea and Febiger, 1979):104.

28. Neal, JB. *Encephalitis: A Clinical Study* (New York: Grune and Stratton, 1942):378-379.

29. See Note 21, pp. 102-103.

30. Ford, F.R. *Diseases of the Nervous System in Infancy, Childhood, and Adolescence,* (Springfield: C.C. Thomas, 1937):349.

31. Lurie, et al. "Late results noted in children presenting post-encephalitic behavior." *American Journal of Psychiatry* 1947;104:178.

32. Baker, AB. "The central nervous system in infectious diseases of childhood." *Postgraduate Medicine* 1949;5:11.

33. Annell, AL. "Pertussis in infancy—a cause of behavioral disorders in children," *Acta Societatis Medicorum Upsaliensis,* XVIII, Supplement 1, (1953):17,33.

34. See Notes 21, pp. 120-121. Also see Notes 27 and 28.

35. See Note 21, pp. 179-181.

36. Bond, ED., et al. *The Treatment of Behavior Disorders Following Encephalitis,* (NY: The Commonwealth Fund, 1931): 14-15.

37. Elliott, FA. "Biological roots of violence," *Proceedings of the American Philosophical Society,* (1983);127(2): 84-93.

38. *The New York Times* (December 5, 1987): B1.

39. Lewis, D. ed. *Vulnerabilities to Delinquency* (NY: SP Medical/Scientific Books, 1981):28.

40. Cowart, VS. "Attention-deficit hyperactivity disorder: physicians helping parents pay more heed," *Journal of American Medical Association* (May 13, 1988);259(18):2647.

41. Thinktwice Global Vaccine Institute. Unsolicited case reports submitted by concerned parents. www.thinktwice.com

42. Ibid.

43. Kalokerinos, A. *Every Second Child Was Doomed to Death—Unless One Dedicated Doctor Could Open His Colleagues' Eyes and Minds* (New Canaan, CT: Keats Pub, 1974).

44. Noble, GR., et al. "Acellular and whole-cell pertussis vaccines in Japan: report of a visit by U.S. scientists." *Journal of the American Medical Association* 1987;257:1351-56.

45. Scott, J. "Report: U.S. slips in fight to cut infant mortality." *Press & Sun Bulletin* (extracted from the *Los Angeles Times,* March 1, 1990).

46. Cherry, JD., et al. "Report of the task force on pertussis and pertussis immunization." *Pediatr* (Jun 1988);81(6):933-84.

47. Walker, AM., et al. "Diphtheria-tetanus-pertussis immunization and sudden infant death syndrome." *Am J Public Health* (August 1987);77(8):945-51.

48. Fine, PE and Chen, RT. "Confounding in studies of adverse reactions to vaccines." *American Journal of Epidemiology* 1992;136(2):121-35.

49. Scheibner, V. *Vaccination: 100 Years of Orthodox Research...* (Blackheath, NSW, Australia: Scheibner Publications, 1993):59-70;225-235.

50. Karlsson, LG and Scheibnerova. "Evidence of the association between non-specific stress syndrome, DPT injections and cot death." Pre-print of a study delivered to the 2nd National Immunisation Conference in Canberra (May 1991).

51. Scheibner, V. ""Evidence of the association between non-specific stress syndrome, DPT injections and cot death." Proceedings of the 2nd National Immunisation Conference in Canberra (May 27-29, 1991).

52. Scheibnerova, V. *Cot Death as Due to Exposure to Non-Specific Stress and General Adaption Syndrome: Its Mechanisms and Prevention* (NSW, Australia: Association for Prevention of Cot Death, October 1990).

53. Torch, WC. "Diphtheria-pertussis-tetanus (DPT) immunization: A potential cause of the sudden infant death syndrome (SIDS)." American Acad of Neurology, 34th Annual Meeting, Apr 25-May 1, 1982. *Neurology* 32(4):pt. 2.

54. See Note 41.

55. Cherry, J.D. "The future use of acellular pertussis vaccines in the U.S." *Vaccine Bulletin* (January 1987):2.

56. Noble, GR., et al. "Acellular and whole-cell pertussis vaccines in Japan: report of a visit by U.S. scientists." *Journal of the American Medical Association* 1987;257:1351-56.

57. Tompson, M. As quoted in: *But Doctor, About That Shot...The Risks of Immunizations...* by Mendelsohn, RS. (Evanston, IL: The People's Doctor Newsletter, Inc., 1988):96.

58. Storsaeter, J., et al. "Mortality and morbidity from invasive bacterial infections during a clinical trial of acellular pertussis vaccines in Sweden." *Pediatric Infectious Disease Journal* 1988;7:637-45.

59. Blennow, M., et al. "Adverse reactions and serologic response to a booster dose of acellular pertussis vaccine in children immunized with acellular or whole-cell vaccine as infants." *Pediatrics* 1989;84:62-67.

60. Fisher, BL. *The Consumer's Guide to Childhood Vaccines.* (Vienna, VA: National Vaccine Information Center, 1997):37.

61. See Note 3.

62. Alderson, M. *International Mortality Statistics* (Wash., DC: Facts on File, 1981):164-65.

63. Ad Hoc Group for the Study of Pertussis Vaccines. "Placebo-controlled trial of two acellular pertussis vaccines in Sweden—protective efficacy and adverse events." *The Lancet* (April 30, 1988):955-60.

64. "License application for pertussis vaccine withdrawn in Sweden." *The Lancet* (January 14, 1989):114.

65. Ibid.

66. Liese, JG., et al. "Efficacy of a two-component acellular pertussis vaccine in infants." *Journal of Pediatric Infectious Disease* 1997;16:1038-44.

67. Vickers, D., et al. "Whole-cell and acellular pertussis vaccination programs and rates of pertussis among infants and young children." *Canadian Med Ass. J.* 2006;175(10):1213-17.

67. Edelman, K., et al. "Immunity to pertussis 5 years after booster immunization during adolescence." *Clinical Infectious Diseases* (May 15, 2007);44:1271-77.

68. Christie, DC., et al. "The 1993 epidemic of pertussis in Cincinnati: resurgence of disease in a highly immunized population of children," *New England Journal of Medicine* (July 7, 1994):16-20.

69. Ewanowich, CA., et al. "Major outbreak of pertussis in Northern Alberta, Canada." *Journal of Clinical Microbiology* (July 1993):1715-25.

70. National Vaccine Information Center. "MedAlerts: access to the U.S. government's Vaccine Adverse Event Reporting System (VAERS)." www.medalerts.org

71. See Note 41.

72. CDC. "Pertussis outbreak—Vermont, 1996." *MMWR* (Sept. 5, 1997);46(35): 822-26.

73. Theodoridou, M., et al. "Pertussis outbreak detected by active surveillance in Cyprus in 2003." *Euro Surveillance* (May 2007);12(5).

74. Moerman, L., et al. "The re-emergence of pertussis in Israel." Israel Vaccine Research Initiative. *Israel Medical Association Journal* (May 2006);8:308-311.

75. Ibid.

76. O'Brien, W. "Hunterdon health department monitors continuing whooping cough outbreak." *My Central Jersey* (January 14, 2009). www.mycentraljersey.com

77. Cherry, JD. "Immunity to pertussis." *Clinical Infectious Diseases* (May 15, 2007); 44:1278.

Measles

What is measles?
Measles is a contagious disease that produces a pink rash all over the body. It is caused by a virus that affects the respiratory system, skin and eyes. The first symptoms appear about 10 days after becoming infected. A fever, cough, and runny nose develop, and the eyes become red, watery and sensitive to light. The fever may reach 105° F (41°C). Small pink spots with gray-white centers occur inside the mouth. A few days later, pink spots break out on the face. The rash then spreads all over the body. Once the rash reaches the feet—in two or three days—the fever drops and the runny nose and cough disappear. The rash on other parts of the body begins to fade, and the infected person starts to feel better.

Antibiotics and drugs do not work to shorten the duration or alleviate the symptoms of measles once it is contracted. Treatment mainly consists of allowing the disease to run its course. However, cool sponge baths and soothing lotions to relieve the itchy rash may be helpful. Drinking lots of liquids to prevent dehydration is recommended as well. The disease confers permanent immunity; the infected person will not contract it again.

Is measles dangerous?
Prior to the 1960s, most children in the U.S. and Canada caught measles. Complications from the disease were unlikely. Previously healthy children usually recovered without incident. However, measles can be dangerous in populations newly exposed to the virus, and in malnourished children living in undeveloped countries. Ear infections, pneumonia, brain damage (subacute sclerosing panencephalitis), and death are some of the possibilities. In advanced countries, measles can be severe when it infects people living in impoverished communities with poor nutrition, sanitation, and inadequate health care. Complications are also more likely when the disease strikes infants, adults, and anyone with a compromised immune system.

Vitamin A and nutrition: Several studies show that when patients with measles are given vitamin A supplements, their complication rates and chances of dying are significantly reduced. Other studies confirm that the wild measles virus has a severe short-term negative effect on immunity and the child's nutritional status, especially vitamin A levels. Mild vitamin A deficiency in children who contract measles has been associated with a higher risk of diarrhea, respiratory disease, and death.[1-5]

In 1987, the *British Medical Journal* published a study conducted on 180 African children with measles. They were randomly divided into two groups. Half of the children received routine treatment. The other children received routine treatment plus 200,000 i.u. of orally administered vitamin A. Mortality rates in the vitamin A group were cut in half. In fact, children under two years of age who did not receive vitamin A were nearly eight times more likely to die.[6] In 1990, the *New England Journal of Medicine* confirmed that vitamin A supplements significantly reduce measles complication and death rates.[7]

Malnutrition is clearly responsible for higher disease complication and death rates.[8] According to Dr. David Morley, infectious disease expert, "Severity of measles is greatest in the developing countries where children have nutritional deficiencies."[9] Dr. Viera Scheibner, vaccine researcher, summarizes the data more succinctly:

"Children in Third World countries need improved vitamin A and general nutritional status, not vaccines."[10]
—**Dr. Viera Scheibner, vaccine researcher**

Fever reducers: Poor nutrition and a vitamin A deficiency are not the only factors known to increase measles complication and mortality rates. Standard treatment protocols may be detrimental as well. For example, when doctors give fever reducers, such as aspirin, to control the rising temperature in measles patients, greater problems are likely. In one study during a measles epidemic in Africa, children were divided into two groups. One group received fever reducers—typical treatment at many hospitals. Mortality was five times greater than in the group that did not receive this treatment. Researchers concluded that "children with the most violent, highly febrile form of the disease actually had the best prognosis."[11]

In another study, 200 children with measles were divided into two groups. Once again, members of one group received aspirin to lower fever. Children who received the aspirin had prolonged illness, more diarrhea, ear infections and respiratory ailments, such as pneumonia, bronchitis and laryngitis, and significantly greater mortality rates.[12] According to Dr. Harold Buttram, who studied the data, "it could be inferred that interference with the natural course of the disease significantly dampened immune responses of the children."[13] Authors of the study noted that the "adverse effect of [fever reducers], which makes the course of the disease longer, facilitates superinfections which give rise to high mortality."[14]

Dr. Robert Mendelsohn agrees that fevers should not be suppressed:

"Doctors do a great disservice to you and your child when they prescribe drugs to reduce his fever... When your child contracts an infection, the fever that accompanies it is a blessing, not a curse... A rising body temperature simply indicates that the process of healing is speeding up. It is something to rejoice over, not to fear."[15]

—**Robert Mendelsohn, MD, pediatrician**

The measles vaccine:

In 1963, both a live-virus shot and an inactivated vaccine were licensed. By the mid-1960s, several measles vaccines were being given to millions of young children in the U.S. In 1967, the inactivated vaccine was removed from the market. By the early 1970s, Canada and many other countries had begun nationwide measles vaccination campaigns. Today, the current measles vaccine is usually provided via MMR, but is available separately.

- Attenuvax—A live-virus vaccine "propagated in chick embryo cell culture." Each dose includes sodium chloride, sodium phosphate, sucrose, sorbitol, hydrolyzed gelatin, glutamate, neomycin, human albumin and fetal bovine serum. Produced by Merck. Given in 2 doses.[16]

Safety

The measles vaccine has a long history of causing serious adverse reactions. The pharmaceutical company that makes the measles vaccine publishes an extensive list of ailments known to have occurred following the shot. Severe afflictions affecting nearly every body system—blood, lymphatic, digestive, cardiovascular, immune, nervous, respiratory, and sensory—have been linked to this "preventive" inoculation. These include: encephalitis, subacute sclerosing panencephalitis (SSPE), Guillain-Barré syndrome, convulsions, seizures, ataxia, ocular palsies, anaphylaxis, angioneurotic edema, bronchial spasms, panniculitis, vasculitis, thrombocytopenia, lymphadenopathy, leukocytosis, pneumonitis, Stevens-Johnson syndrome, erythema multiforme, urticaria, deafness, otitis media, retinitis, optic neuritis, rash, fever, dizziness, headache, and death.[17,18]

Can the measles vaccine cause BRAIN DAMAGE?

Subacute sclerosing panencephalitis (SSPE) is a slow, progressive disease that begins with mental decline and muscle spasms, then advances over months or years to convulsions, coma, and death. It was first recorded following measles vaccine in 1968, shortly after this shot was introduced.[19]

The following year, a federal SSPE registry was established to document the growing number of cases being reported.[20] Shortly thereafter, the *Journal of the American Medical Association* published an extensive paper on this disturbing new trend.[21] The U.S. National Institutes of Health considers SSPE a delayed or "late" complication of measles, and reports that this slow virus infection occurs "an average of 7 years after initial exposure."[22] Today, children vaccinated with measles (or MMR) continue to run the risk of contracting SSPE. For example, the following case report refers to a healthy 13-year-old girl who received MMR and developed SSPE:

▸ "The child verbalized little and was socially inappropriate; her memory and thinking abilities were impaired. She grew progressively worse, and added myoclonic jerks of the upper limbs, with depressed tendon reflexes."[23]

Other neurological disorders following measles vaccination are well documented in the medical literature. For example, the Medical Research Council in Great Britain tested the new measles vaccine and discovered that vaccinated children had convulsions at more than six times the rate in unvaccinated children.[24] Several scientific journals have published data on encephalitis (inflammation of the brain) and Guillain-Barré syndrome (paralysis) following measles vaccination as well.[25-35]

The measles vaccine and BLEEDING DISORDERS:

Thrombocytopenia, a blood disease resulting in spontaneous bleeding, is a well-known adverse reaction to the measles vaccine. In one study, researchers noted that 86 percent of vaccinated individuals experienced an extreme drop in platelet levels needed for clotting blood.[36] During the 1970s, 1980s, 1990s, and 2000s, wherever measles vaccine campaigns were enforced, including in Sweden, Canada, Germany, Finland, France, and Great Britain, new cases of thrombocytopenia were reported.[37-45] In the United States, the Vaccine Safety Committee officially acknowledged thrombocytopenia as a serious adverse reaction to the measles vaccine.[46]

Can the measles vaccine suppress the IMMUNE SYSTEM?

Studies have shown that the measles vaccine depresses the ability of disease-fighting lymphocytes to perform their duties. They dramatically decline in number after measles vaccination.[47,48] Dr. Richard Moskowitz, former president of the National Center for Homeopathy, offers a possible explanation. He believes that the weakened measles virus injected directly into the bloodstream may cause antibodies to inhibit an acute inflammatory response to the virus. Months or years later, during periods of stress, they may attack the body's own cells resulting in an autoimmune crisis.[49]

Moskowitz surmised that the unnatural process of vaccination may bring about the "far less curable chronic diseases of the present."[50] Also, "these illnesses may be more serious than the original disease, involving deeper structures [and] more vital organs."[51] Dr. Moskowitz elaborated:

> *"The permanent immunity acquired in recovering from the natural disease [measles] represents a net gain for the total health of the human race. 'True' or lifelong immunity of this type cannot be ascribed to the measles vaccine.... Because the vaccinated individual has no obvious way of getting rid of the virus, the technical feat of antibody synthesis presumably represents, at most, a memory of **chronic infection**. It makes no sense to claim that vaccines render us 'immune' to viruses if in fact they weaken our ability to expel them, and force us to harbor them permanently. Indeed, my concern and growing conviction is that such a carrier state tends to compromise our ability to respond to other infections. In that sense, vaccines must themselves be regarded as immunosuppressive."[52]*
>
> **—Richard Moskowitz, MD**

The measles vaccine and BOWEL DISEASE:

In 1995, *The Lancet* published a landmark study showing that babies vaccinated with measles are at greater risk than unvaccinated children to develop inflammatory bowel disease later in life. Scientists believe that the vaccine, which contains attenuated measles virus, provokes the immune system into attacking its own intestinal cells. The study found one case of inflammatory bowel disease for every 142 people vaccinated against measles. In fact, people who received the measles vaccine were 2½ times more likely to develop ulcerative colitis and three times more likely to develop Crohn's disease when compared to unvaccinated controls.[53]

The measles vaccine and SEVERE ALLERGIC REACTIONS:

Some people are hypersensitive to ingredients in the measles vaccine, such as egg proteins (from the chick embryo cell cultures used to propagate the measles virus), neomycin (an antibiotic) and hydrolyzed gelatin. This can lead to anaphylaxis, an extreme allergic reaction that may cause the victim's heart to stop or throat to swell cutting off oxygen, painful cramps, seizures, shock, collapse, and death. Numerous reports of anaphylaxis after measles (and MMR) vaccination have been documented.[54-59]

The measles vaccine and SENSORY DISORDERS:

The potential for eye damage and hearing loss following measles (or MMR) vaccination is also well documented in the medical literature.[60-65]

Measles Vaccine Reaction: Congressional Testimony

The following excerpt is from a statement made by a distraught mother testifying before the U.S. Congress:

"My name is Wendy Scholl. I reside in the state of Florida with my husband, Gary, and three daughters, Stacy, Holly, and Jackie. Let me stress that all three of our daughters were born healthy, normal babies. I am here to tell of Stacy's reaction to the measles vaccine...where according to the medical profession, anything within 7 to 10 days after the vaccine to do with neurological sequelae or seizures or brain damage fits a measles reaction....

At 16 months old, Stacy received her measles shot. She was a happy, healthy, normal baby, typical, curious, playful until the 10th day after her shot when I walked into her room to find her laying in her crib, flat on her stomach, her head twisted to one side. Her eyes were glassy and affixed. She was panting, struggling to breathe. Her small body lay in a pool of blood that hung from her mouth. It was a terrifying sight, yet at that point I didn't realize that my happy, bouncing baby was never to be the same.

When we arrived at the emergency room, Stacy's temperature was 107 degrees. The first four days of Stacy's hospital stay she battled for life. She was in a coma and had kidney failure. Her lungs filled with fluid and she had ongoing seizures.

Her diagnosis was 'post-vaccinal encephalitis' and her prognosis was grave. She was paralyzed on her left side, prone to seizures, had visual problems. However, we were told by doctors we were extremely lucky. I didn't feel lucky. We were horrified that this vaccine which was given only to ensure that she would have a safer childhood, almost killed her. I didn't know that the possibility of this type of reaction even existed. But now, it is our reality."[66]

Efficacy

According to the vaccine manufacturer, "Extensive clinical trials have demonstrated that Attenuvax is highly immunogenic.... A single injection of the vaccine has been shown to induce measles inhibition antibodies in 97% or more of susceptible persons." Also, "Efficacy of measles vaccine was established in a series of double-blind controlled field trials which demonstrated a high degree of protective efficacy."[67] However, nearly all of these so-called "extensive clinical trials" and "series of double-blind controlled field trials" are either unavailable for review because the data is "unpublished" (sealed by the manufacturer) or the available data refers to studies conducted in the 1960s—about 50 years ago—long before the current measles vaccine, Attenuvax (and MMR), became available.[68-75]

During the pre-vaccine era, measles was a common childhood illness. Nearly everyone contracted it by the age of 10 and developed permanent immunity as a result. After the vaccine was introduced, measles declined to an average of 3000 cases per year in the 1980s, and even fewer cases per year during the 1990s and 2000s.[76] However, a significant decline in measles began long before the vaccine was introduced. From 1958 to 1962, the number of cases toppled by 38 percent. The measles death rate tumbled on its own even more. In 1900, there were 13.3 measles deaths in the United States per 100,000 population. By 1955, eight years *before* the first measles shot, the death rate had declined by 98 percent to .03 deaths per 100,000. England experienced a similar decline in measles cases and the measles death rate *before* the vaccine was introduced.[77]

What is HERD IMMUNITY? Can it be achieved?

Authorities believe that if a certain percentage of people in society are immune to a disease, epidemics will not occur.[78] In 1991, the CDC concluded that measles outbreaks can be avoided if 70 to 80 percent of two-year-olds in inner cities are vaccinated.[79] A 1992 study published in the *Journal of the American Medical Association* also concluded that "immunization coverage of two-year-olds of 80 percent or less may be sufficient to prevent sustained measles outbreaks in urban communities."[80] Other authorities acknowledge that "the level of coverage required to prevent transmission of measles is unknown."[81] Outbreaks have occurred in communities where 97 percent of the population was "protected."[82] Thus, after examining 320 scientific works from around the world, 180 European medical doctors concluded that...

"The eradication of measles...would today appear to be an unrealistic goal."[83]
—**Conclusion reached by 180 European medical doctors**

Professor D. Levy of Johns Hopkins University also weighed the odds of eradicating measles with mass immunization campaigns and concluded that if current practices [of suppressing natural immunity] continue, by the year 2050 a large part of the population will be at risk and "there could in theory be over 25,000 fatal cases of measles in the USA."[84]

The measles vaccine does not confer permanent immunity—one reason eradication of the disease is so elusive. Epidemics regularly occur in vaccinated populations. Dr. William Atkinson, senior epidemiologist with the CDC, admitted that...

"Measles transmission has been clearly documented among vaccinated persons. In some large outbreaks...over 95 percent of cases have a history of vaccination."[85]

—**William Atkinson, MD, Senior Epidemiologist, CDC**

According to the World Health Organization, the odds are about 15 times greater that measles will strike those vaccinated against the disease than those who are left alone.[86] The medical literature contains many large-scale examples of documented vaccine failures. For example, in 1988, 69 percent of all school-aged children in the U.S. who contracted measles were previously vaccinated against the disease.[87] In 1989, 58 percent of all school-age measles cases in Canada, and 89 percent of all school-age measles cases in the U.S. were previously vaccinated.[88,89] In 1995, 56 percent of all measles cases in the U.S. occurred in people who were previously vaccinated.[90] In 2000, Nepal had a measles outbreak in which *all* (100 percent) of the people who caught measles were vaccinated against the disease.[91] In 2003, there was a measles outbreak in a Pennsylvania school with 99 percent "herd immunity" from vaccination; 67 percent of the measles cases occurred in students fully vaccinated against measles.[92] In 2007, Saudi Arabia had a measles outbreak; 62 percent of the cases were in people vaccinated against measles.[93] Today, the CDC and WHO continue to document cases of measles in previously vaccinated individuals.

The measles vaccine shifted the disease to riskier age groups:
The measles vaccine dramatically altered distribution of the disease by shifting incidence rates from age-groups unlikely to experience problems (children 5 to 9 years old) to age-groups most likely to suffer from severe complications (infants, teenagers, and adults). In 1963, *before* the measles vaccine was introduced, it was extremely rare for infants to develop measles. This was because their mothers had contracted measles naturally as children and developed protective antibodies that were passed on to their babies during birth. These babies were secure from measles for the first 15 months of life. However, by the 1990s, more than 25 percent of all measles cases were now occurring in infants. CDC officials admit that this situation is likely to get worse, and attribute it to the growing number of mothers who were vaccinated. Fewer mothers now have natural immunity.[94-96]

Pediatrics published a study showing that infants of mothers born after 1963 are 7½ times more likely to contract measles than infants of mothers born earlier.[97] In 2000, the *Journal of Medical Virology* published a study that ominously noted that...

"With an increasing proportion of mothers being vaccinated, the number of infants susceptible to resistant wild-type viruses may increase dramatically."[98]
—Conclusion reached in the *Journal of Medical Virology*

Today, a higher percentage of teenagers and adults are suffering from measles. *Before* the measles vaccine was introduced, just 3 percent of cases were in persons 15 years and older. *After* the vaccine was introduced, 26 percent of all cases occurred in persons 15 years and older.[99] By 1999, the CDC confirmed that at least 50 percent of all measles cases were still occurring in high-risk age groups that were not susceptible to measles during the pre-vaccine era.[100]

The risk of measles-related pneumonia and liver abnormalities is greater in the adolescent and young adult age-groups. According to a study published in the *Journal of Infectious Diseases,* such complications have increased by as much as 20 percent.[101] The risk of death from measles is also much higher for infants and adults than for children.

Notes

1. Oomen, APC. "Clinical experience of hypovitamine A." *Federation Proceedings* 1958; 17:111-124.

2. Wilson, D., et al. "Infection and nutritional status. III. The effect of measles on nitrogen metabolism in children." *Amer J of Clinical Nutrition* 1961;9:154-58.

3. Sommer, A., et al. "Increased risk of respiratory disease and diarrhea in children with pre-existing mild vitamin A deficiency." *Amer J of Clinical Nutrition* 1984;40:1090-95.

4. Sommer, A., et al. "Impact of vitamin A supplementation on childhood mortality: a randomized clinical trial." *The Lancet* 1986;1:1169-73.

5. Frieden, TR., et al. "Vitamin A levels and severity of measles: New York City." *American Journal of Diseases of Children* 1992; 146:182-86.

6. Barclay, AJG., et al. "Vitamin A supplements and mortality related to measles: a randomised clinical trial." *British Medical Journal* (January 31, 1987):294-96.

7. Keusch, GT. "Vitamin A supplements—too good to be true." *New England Journal of Medicine* (October 4, 1990):986.

8. Krishnamurthy, KA., et al. "Measles a dangerous disease: a study of 1000 cases in Madurai." *Indian Pediatr* 1974:267-71.

9. Morley, D. "Severe measles: some unanswered questions." *Reviews of Infectious Diseases* (May/June 1983):460-62.

10. Scheibner, V. *Vaccination: 100 Years of Orthodox Research Shows that Vaccines Represent a Medical Assault on the Immune System.* (Australia: Scheibner Pub., 1993):92.

11. Witsenburg, BC. "Measles mortality and therapy," pp. 26-27. From an abstract of a 1967-1968 measles epidemic study conducted in Ghana.

12. Ahmady, AS., et al. "The adverse effects of antipyretics in measles." *Indian Pediatrics* (January 1981):49-52.

13. Buttram, Harold. In a foreword to *Vaccines: Are They Really Safe and Effective?* by Neil Z. Miller. (Santa Fe, NM: New Atlantean Press, 2008):10.

14. See Note 12.

15. Mendelsohn, R. *How to Raise a Healthy Child...In Spite of Your Doctor.* (Ballantine Books, 1987):80-81; 237-238.

16. Merck & Co., Inc. "Attenuvax® (Measles Virus Vaccine Live)." Product insert from the vaccine manufacturer (Issued: February 2006).

17. Ibid.

18. National Vaccine Information Center. "MedAlerts: access to the U.S. government's Vaccine Adverse Event Reporting System (VAERS)." www.medalerts.org

19. Schneck, S.A. "Vaccination with measles and central nervous system disease." *Neurology* 1968;18 (part 2):79-82.

20. Institute of Medicine. *Adverse Events Associated with Childhood Vaccines: Evidence Bearing on Causality.* (Washington, DC: National Acad. Press, 1994).

21. Jabbour, JT., et al. "Epidemiology of subacute sclerosing panencephalitis (SSPE)." *Journal of the American Medical Association* 1972;220:959-62.

22. National Institutes of Health. "The search for health: eliminating measles." *U.S. Department of Health and Human Services* (April 1983).

23. Belgamwar, RB., et al. "Measles, mumps, rubella vaccine induced subacute sclerosing panencephalitis." *Journal of the Indian Medical Association* 1997;95(11):594.

24. Miller, CL. "Convulsions after measles vaccination." *The Lancet* (July 23, 1983):215.

25. Landrigan, PJ., et al. "Neurological disorders following live measles-virus vaccination." *Journal of the American Medical Association* 1973;223(13):1459-62.

26. Beale, AJ. "Measles vaccines." *Proc of the Royal Soc. of Med.* 1974;67:1116-1119.

27. Roden, AT. "Fits following immunization." *Proc of the Royal Soc of Med* 1974;67:24.

28. Jagdis, F., et al. "Encephalitis after administration of live measles vaccine." *Journal of the Canadian Medical Association* (April 19, 1975);112(8):972-75.

29. Hirayama, M. "Measles vaccines used in Japan." *Rev. of Infectious Dis.* 1983;5:495-503.

30. Pollock, TM., et al. "A 7-year survey of disorders attributed to vaccination in NW Thames Region." *The Lancet* 1983;1:753-57.

31. Jorch, G. et al. "Coincidence of virus encephalitis and measles-mumps vaccination." *Monatsschr Kinderheilkd* 1984; 132(5):299-300.

32. Martinon-Torres, F., et al. "Self-limited acute encephalopathy related to measles component of viral triple vaccine." *Rev Neur* (May 1-15, 1999);28(9):881-2.

33. Grose, C., et al. "Guillain-Barré syndrome following administration of live measles vaccine." *American Journal of Medicine* 1976;60:441-43.

34. Norrby, R. "Polyradiculitis in connection with vaccination against morbilli, parotitis and rubella." *Lakartidningen* 1984;81:1636-37.

35. Morris, K., et al. "Guillain-Barré syndrome after measles, mumps, and rubella vaccine." *The Lancet* 1994; 343:60.

36. Oski, FA., et al. "Effect of live measles vaccine on the platelet count." *New England Journal of Medicine* 1966;265:352-56.

37. Bottiger, M., et al. "Swedish experience of two dose vaccination programme aiming at eliminating measles, mumps, and rubella." *British Medical Journal* 1987;295:1264-67.

38. Koch, J. et al. "Adverse events temporally associated with immunizing agents—1987 report." *Canada Diseases Weekly Report* 1989;15:151-58.

39. Fescharek, R., et al. "Measles-mumps vaccination in the FRG: an empirical analysis after 14 years of use. II. Tolerability and analysis of spontaneously reported side effects." *Vaccine* 1990;8:446-56.

40. Nieminen, U., et al. "Acute thrombocytopenic purpura following measles, mumps and rubella vaccination: A report on 23 patients." *Acta Paediatrica* 1993; 82:267-70.

41. Farrington, P., et al. "A new method for active surveillance of adverse events from diphtheria/tetanus/pertussis and measles/mumps/rubella vaccines." *Lancet* 1995;345:567-69.

42. Jonville-Bera, AP., et al. "Thrombocytopenic purpura after measles, mumps, and rubella vaccination: a retrospective survey by the French Regional Pharmaco-vigilance Centres and Pasteur-Merieux Serums et Vaccins." *Pediatr Infect Dis J* 1996;15:44-48.

43. Beeler, J. et al. "Thrombocytopenia after immunization with measles vaccines: review of the Vaccine Adverse Events Reporting System 1990-94." *The Pediatric Infectious Disease Journal* 1996;15:88-90.

44. CDC. "Update: Vaccine Side Effects, Adverse Reactions, Contraindications, and Precautions. Recommendations of the Advisory Committee on Immunization Practices (ACIP)." *MMWR* (September 6, 1996); 45(RR-12):1-35.

45. See Note 18.

46. See Note 20.

47. Hirsch, RL., et al. "Measles virus vaccination of measles seropositive individuals suppresses lymphocyte proliferation and chemotactic factor production." *Clinical Immunology and Immunopathology* 1981;21:341-50.

48. Nicholson, JKA., et al. "The effect of measles-rubella vaccination on lymphocyte populations and subpopulations in HIV-infected and healthy individuals." *Journal of Acquired Immune Deficiency Syndromes* 1992;5:528-537.

49. Moskowitz, R. "The case against immunizations." *Journal of the American Institute of Homeopathy* 1983;76:7-25.

50. Moskowitz, R. "Immunizations: a dissenting view." *Dissent in Medicine—Nine Doctors Speak Out* (Contemporary Books, 1985):133-66.

51. Moskowitz, R. "Immunizations: the other side." *Mothering* (Spring 1984):33-4.

52. Moskowitz, R. "Vaccination: A sacrament of modern medicine." *Vaccination: The Issue of Our Times* (Mothering Magazine, 1997):169.

53. Thompson, NP., Wakefield, AJ, et al. "Is measles vaccination a risk factor for inflammatory bowel disease?" *The Lancet* 1995;345:1071-1074.

54. Aukrust, L., et al. "Severe hypersensitivity or intolerance reactions to measles vaccine in 6 children: clinical & immunological studies." *Allergy* 1980;35(7):581-87.

55. McEwen, J. "Early-onset reaction after measles vaccination: further Australian reports." *Medical Journal of Australia* 1983;2:503-505.

56. Koch, J., et al. "Adverse events temporally associated with immunizing agents—1987 report." *Canada Diseases Weekly Report* 1989;15:151-58.

57. Kelso, JM., et al. "Anaphylaxis to measles, mumps, and rubella vaccine mediated by IgE to gelatin." *J Allergy Clin Immunol* 1993;91:867-72.

58. Sakaguchi, M., et al. "IgE antibody to gelatin in children with immediate-type reactions to measles and mumps vaccines." *J Allergy Clin Immunol* 1995;96:563-65.

59. See Note 18.

60. Kazarian, EL., et al. "Optic neuritis complicating measles, mumps, and rubella vaccination." *Amer J of Ophthalmology* 1978;86:544-47.

61. Marshall, GS., et al. "Diffuse retinopathy following measles, mumps, and rubella vaccination." *Pediatrics* 1985;76:989-991.

62. Brodsky, L., et al. "Sensorineural hearing loss following live measles virus vaccination." *International J of Pediatric Otorhinolaryngology* 1985;10:159-63.

63. Nabe-Nielsen, J., et al. "Unilateral deafness as a complication of the mumps, measles, and rubella vaccination." *British Medical Journal* 1988;297:489.

64. Hulbert, TV., et al. "Bilateral hearing loss after measles and rubella vaccination in an adult." *New England Journal of Medicine* 1991;325:134.

65. Stewart, BJA., et al. "Reports of sensorineural deafness after measles, mumps, and rubella immunisation." *Archives of Diseases of Childhood* 1993;69:153-54.

66. Hearings Before the Subcommittee on Health and the Environment: Vaccine Injury Compensation. 98th Congress, 2nd Session (December 19, 1984):110.

67. See Note 16.

68. Unpublished data: Files of Merck Research Laboratories.

69. Studies conducted under the direction of Dr. Conrado Ristori, National Health Service, Santiago, Chile (Unpublished Data).

70. Studies conducted under the direction of Dr. Victor Villarejos, Louisiana State University International Center of Medical Research and Training, San Jose, Costa Rica (Unpublished Data).

71. Hilleman, MR., et al. "Development and evaluation of the Moraten measles virus vaccine, *Journal of the American Medical Association* 1968;206(3):587-590.

72. Swartz, T., et al. "A comparative study of four live measles vaccines in Israel." *Bull. WHO* 1968;39:285-292.

73. Krugman, S., et al. "Comparison of two further attenuated live measles-virus vaccines." *Amer. J. Dis. Child* (February 1969);117:137-138.

74. Cutts, FT., et al. "Principles of measles control." *Bull WHO* 1991;69(1):1-7.

75. See Note 16.

76. CDC. "Summary of notifiable diseases, U.S., 1993." *MMWR* 1994;42(53).

77. Alderson, M. *International Mortality Statistics* (Washington, DC: Facts on File, 1981):182-183.

78. Cherry, JD. "The 'new' epidemiology of measles and rubella." *Hospital Practice* (July 1980):50.

79. CDC. "Measles vaccination levels among selected groups of preschool-aged children —USA." *MMWR* 1991;40:36-39.

80. Schlenker, TL., et al. "Measles herd immunity: the association of attack rats with immunization rates in preschool children." *JAMA* 1992;267(6):826.

81. Gold, E. "Current progress in measles eradication in the U.S." *Infect Med* 1997;14(4): 297-300,310.

82. Ibid.

83. Albonico, H., Klein, P., et al. "The immunization campaign against measles, mumps and rubella—coercion leading to a realm of uncertainty: medical objections to a continued MMR immunization campaign in Switzerland." *J of Anthroposophic Medicine* 1992;9(1).

84. Levy, D. "The future of measles in highly immunized populations." *American Journal of Epidemiology* 1984;120:39-47.

85. FDA. "FDA workshop to review warnings, use instructions, and precautionary information [on vaccines]." (Rockland, Maryland: FDA, September 18, 1992):27.

86. See Note 15, p. 238.

87. CDC. "Measles." *MMWR* 1989;38:329-330.

88. CDC. "Measles—Quebec." *MMWR* 1989;38:329-30.

89. Resnick, SK. "Should you get vaccinated against measles?" *Natural Health* (January/February 1992):30.

90. CDC. "U.S. Childhood Immunization Update: Measles." (March 1997). Also see Note 81.

91. Khan, JN., et al. "Measles outbreak in a vaccinated population in Dhankutta." *Nepal Med Coll J* 2003;5(1):16-7.

92. Yeung, LF., et al. "A limited measles outbreak in a highly vaccinated U.S. boarding school." *Pediatrics* 2005;116(6):1287-1291.

93. Jahan, S., et al. "Measles outbreak in Qassim, Saudi Arabia 2007." *J of Public Health* 2008;30(4):384-90.

94. CDC. "Measles—United States, 1999." *MMWR* 2000;49(25):557-560.

95. Papania, M., et al. "Increased susceptibility to measles in infants in the United States." American Academy of Pediatrics (November 1999);104(5):e59.

96. CDC. Cited in Haney, DQ. "Wave of infant measles stems from '60s vaccinations." *Albuquerque Journal* (November 23, 1992):B3.

97. CDC. "Babies of vaccinated moms more susceptible to measles." *Pediatrics* (November 1999).

98. Klingele, M., et al. "Resistance of recent measles virus wild-type isolates to antibody-mediated neutralization by vaccinees with antibody." *J of Medical Virology* 2000;62:91-98.

99. See Note 78, p. 51.

100. CDC. "Measles—United States, 1999." *MMWR* 2000;49(25):557-560.

101. Rizetto, M., et al. *Journal of Infectious Diseases* (Jan 1982):18-22.

Mumps

What is mumps?

Mumps is a contagious disease caused by a virus. The illness begins with a fever, headache, muscle aches, and fatigue. Salivary glands beneath the ears along the jaw line become swollen. In some instances, testicles, ovaries, and female breasts may also swell. Treatment mainly consists of allowing the disease to run its course. Medical intervention is seldom required. Symptoms usually disappear within a week. The disease confers permanent immunity; the infected person will not contract it again.

Is mumps dangerous?

Mumps is a relatively harmless disease when it is experienced in childhood. Complications are uncommon but can be much more severe when they occur in teenagers and adults. For example, orchitis (inflammation of the testes) occurs in about 20 percent of mumps cases in post-pubescent males. This has caused some people to claim mumps will prevent a man from fathering children. However, orchitis usually affects only one testicle; sterility from the ailment is extremely rare. Mumps has also been associated with transient meningitis, temporary hearing loss, and inflammation of the ovaries. Full recovery without complications usually follows in 3 to 4 days. Permanent harm from mumps, including death, is rare.[1-3]

The mumps vaccine:

In 1967, the first mumps vaccine was licensed in the United States. It was put into general use during the 1970s. Today, several mumps vaccines are available throughout the world using different strains of the live mumps virus (i.e., the Jeryl Lynn, Urabe, Leningrad-Zagreb, or Leningrad-3 strains). The current mumps vaccine is usually provided in conjunction with the measles and rubella vaccines (via MMR), but is available separately.

• Mumpsvax—A preparation of the Jeryl Lynn strain of mumps virus "propagated in chick embryo cell culture." This vaccine also contains sodium chloride, sodium phosphate, sucrose, sorbitol, glutamate, hydrolyzed gelatin (an animal protein usually derived from cows or pigs), neomycin (an antibiotic), human albumin, and fetal bovine serum. Produced by Merck. Given in 2 doses.[4]

Contracting Mumps in Childhood may Provide Benefits

Childhood diseases can have a *favorable* effect on the child's immune system. When children overcome illnesses on their own, they build resistance against other diseases in later life. For example, several studies show that women are less likely to develop ovarian cancer if they have had mumps in childhood.[5-8] This may be the best reason several European doctors proclaimed, "there is no plausible medical reason...to immunize girls against mumps."[9]

Safety

The drug company that produces and distributes the mumps vaccine publishes an extensive list of ailments known to have occurred following the mumps (or MMR) shot. These include aseptic meningitis, encephalitis, diabetes mellitus, orchitis (inflammation of one or both of the testicles), parotitis (the technical name for mumps), thrombocytopenia (a serious blood disorder), arthritis, otitis media, optic neuritis, anaphylaxis, Guillain-Barré syndrome, pancreatitis, convulsions, seizures, and death.[10,11]

The mumps vaccine and MENINGITIS:
Several studies have linked the mumps vaccine to meningitis (inflammation of the protective membranes covering the brain and spinal cord) and other complications of the nervous system. For example, the Institute of Medicine showed that the mumps vaccine-virus strain could be isolated from neurologically impaired patients following vaccination. Aseptic meningitis was "officially" recognized as resulting from the mumps vaccine.[12] European scientists published data showing that mumps meningitis had an attack rate of 1 case per every 1000 children vaccinated.[13] Japanese researchers reported higher incidence rates: 1 case per 2000 doses in one study, and 6 cases per 2000 doses in another study.[14,15] *The Lancet* published data showing that all the cases of "lymphocytic meningitis" and mumps meningitis occurred between 17 and 34 days following MMR vaccination.[16]

The mumps vaccine and DIABETES:
Several peer-reviewed journals—including the *Journal of Pediatrics*— documented the onset of juvenile diabetes following mumps vaccination.[17-20] The *New England Journal of Medicine* confirmed that viruses can trigger diabetes.[21] (The mumps and MMR vaccines contain live viruses.) In Europe, 180 doctors issued a warning that the mumps vaccine "can trigger diabetes, which only becomes apparent months after vaccination."[22]

Mumps Vaccine: VAERS Case Reports

▸328170: A 14-month-old baby received the mumps vaccine and one hour later developed an itchy rash in the genital area.

▸57640: A 15-month-old baby received the mumps vaccine and one week later developed encephalitis, convulsions, and went into a coma.

▸305048: A two-year-old boy received the mumps vaccine and three weeks later was diagnosed with mumps.

▸102927: A four-year-old boy received the mumps vaccine and developed diabetes three to six months later.

▸59696: A five-year-old boy received the mumps vaccine and one week later was hospitalized for Schoenlein-Henoch purpura and severe gastroenteritis.

▸205391: A five-year-old boy developed "serious meningitis" nine days after receiving the mumps vaccine.[23]

The mumps (and MMR) vaccine can cause adverse reactions in adults as well:

"I had an MMR (measles, mumps and rubella) vaccine at age 36 because I was returning to school and needed it or I couldn't enroll. Within days of the vaccine, I developed mumps-like symptoms that lasted six months: lump in the throat, swelling, difficulty swallowing. Then I developed a rare, recurrent condition called subacute thyroiditis, which causes swelling of throat tissue, lungs and thyroid, and disrupts your entire system. The severe, scary symptoms include heart palpitations, swallowing difficulty and shallow breathing. I have landed in the emergency room four times. I am convinced the vaccine had something to do with this rare condition because they have concluded it is viral-based, and they have taken tissue from my thyroid and cultivated mumps from it!"[24]
—**Adult victim of the mumps (MMR) vaccine**

Efficacy

Prior to the mumps vaccine, most children under 10 years of age contracted the disease. During the early 1980s, there were about 4000 cases per year.[25] However, outbreaks of mumps often occur in vaccinated populations. For example, in one high school outbreak 94 percent of all cases with known vaccination status occurred in previously vaccinated students. In fact, the vaccinated teenagers were more than twice as likely as the unvaccinated teens to contract the disease.[26] In other outbreaks, up to 99 percent of all cases were in previously vaccinated people.[27]

By 1995, there were less than 1,000 reported cases in the United States. Similar figures were reported in the United Kingdom. However, in 2004 and 2005, there was an epidemic of more than 70,000 cases of mumps in the U.K., despite an 82 percent vaccination rate. More than 30 percent of the cases were in previously vaccinated persons.[28] In 2006, 11 states reported 2,597 cases of mumps; 74 percent of the cases had been fully vaccinated with MMR—they had received the recommended two doses of the mumps vaccine—and 92 percent had received at least one shot of the supposedly "protective" mumps vaccine. Only 8 percent of cases occurred in unvaccinated people.[29] In 2010, the CDC reported on a mumps outbreak affecting nearly 2,000 people. At least 93 percent of the cases in youth 7-18 years of age—the age group with the majority of cases—were previously vaccinated against mumps; 85% had received the recommended two doses. Only 7 percent of cases occurred in unvaccinated people.[30,31]

The mumps vaccine shifted the disease to older age groups:
Years ago, the eminent pediatrician, Dr. Robert Mendelsohn, noted with great foresight that if immunity from the mumps vaccine proves to be temporary...

"There is an open question whether, when your child is immunized against mumps at 15 months and escapes this disease in childhood, he may suffer more serious consequences when he contracts it as an adult. If the mumps immunization is given to protect adult males from orchitis—not to prevent children from getting mumps—it would seem reasonable to administer it only to those males who haven't developed natural immunity by the time they reach puberty. They would then be more certain of protection as adults. All girls and countless boys would thus avoid the potential consequences of a hazardous vaccine."[32]
—Robert Mendelsohn, MD, pediatrician

As Dr. Mendelsohn foresaw, the mumps vaccine did indeed shift incidence rates of the disease from young children to teens and adults. Mumps in young children is a mild, benign disease. It is a more serious disease when contracted by older age groups. Before the mumps vaccine, most children caught the disease. From 1967 to 1971, before this shot was put into general use, 92 percent of all cases occurred in persons 14 years of age or younger. Just 8 percent of cases occurred in persons 15 years of age or older.[33] By 2004, more than 79 percent of all cases were contracted by older persons. Today, teens and adults continue to contract mumps at greater rates than before the vaccine was introduced.[34]

Notes

1. CDC Fact Sheet. "Facts about mumps for adults." *National Coalition for Adult Immunization* (April 2000).
2. Diodati, C. *Immunization: History, Ethics, Law and Health.* (Windsor, Ontario, Canada: Integral Aspects Inc., 1999):113.
3. McKinley Health Center. "Mumps vaccine." *U. of Illinois* (October 5, 1998).
4. Merck & Co., Inc. "Mumpsvax® (Mumps Virus Vaccine Live) Jeryl Lynn Strain." Product insert from the vaccine manufacturer (Issued: September 2002).
5. West, R. "Epidemiologic study of malignancies of the ovaries." *Cancer* 1966;19:1001-1007.
6. Wynder, E., et al. "Epidemiology of cancer of the ovary." *Cancer* 1969;23:352.
7. Newhouse, M., et al. "A case control study of carcinoma of the ovary." *Brit J Prev Soc Med* 1977;31:148-53.
8. McGowan, L., et al. "The woman at risk from developing ovarian cancer." *Gynecol Oncol* 1979;7:325-344.
9. Albonico, H., et al. "The immunization campaign against measles, mumps and rubella—coercion leading to a realm of uncertainty: medical objections to a continued MMR immunization campaign in Switzerland." *Journal of Anthroposophic Medicine* 1992;9(1).
10. Merck & Co., Inc. "M-M-R®II (Measles, Mumps, and Rubella Virus Vaccine Live)." Product insert from the vaccine manufacturer (Issued: December 2007).
11. See Note 4.
12. Institute of Medicine. *Adverse Events Associated with Childhood Vaccines: Evidence Bearing on Causality.* (Washington, DC: National Acad. Press, 1994).
13. Cizman, M., et al. "Aseptic meningitis after vaccination against measles and mumps." *Pediatric Infectious Disease Journal* 1989;8:302-308.
14. Sugiura, A., et al. "Aseptic meningitis as a complication of mumps vaccination." *J of Pediatr Infect Dis* 1991;10:209-213.
15. Fujinaga, T., et al. "A prefecture-wide survey of mumps meningitis associated with measles, mumps and rubella vaccine." *J of Pediatr Infect Dis* 1991;10:204-209.
16. Colville, A., et al. "Mumps meningitis and measles, mumps, and rubella vaccine." *The Lancet* 1992; 340:786.
17. Sultz, HA., et al. "Is mumps virus an etiologic factor in juvenile diabetes mellitus?" *Journal of Pediatrics* 1975;86:654-656.
18. Otten, A., et al. "Mumps, mumps vaccination, islet cell antibodies and the first manifestation of diabetes mellitus type I." *Behring Inst. Mitteilungen* 1984; 75:83-88.
19. Helmke, K., et al. "Islet cell antibodies and the development of diabetes mellitus in relation to mumps infection and mumps vaccination." *Diabetologia* 1986;29:30-33.
20. Pawlowski, B., et al. "Mumps vaccination and type-1 diabetes." *Deutsche Medizinische Wochenschrift* 1991;116:635.
21. Maclaren, N., et al. "Is insulin-dependent diabetes mellitus environmentally induced?" *New England Journal of Medicine* 1992;327:348-349.
22. See Note 9.
23. National Vaccine Information Center. "MedAlerts: access to the U.S. government's Vaccine Adverse Event Reporting System (VAERS)." www.medalerts.org
24. Thinktwice Global Vaccine Institute. Unsolicited case reports submitted by concerned parents. www.thinktwice.com
25. CDC. "Summary of notifiable diseases, United States, 1993." *MMWR* 1994; 42(53).
26. Fiumara, NJ., et al. "Mumps outbreak in Westwood, Massachusetts—1981." *MMWR* 1982; 33(29):421-430.

27. Briss, PA., et al. "Sustained transmission of mumps in a highly vaccinated population: assessment of vaccine failure and waning vaccine-induced immunity." *Journal of Infectious Diseases* 1994;169:77-82.

28. Savage, E., et al. "Mumps epidemic—United Kingdom, 2004-2005." *JAMA* (April 12, 2006);295(14):1636-37.

29. CDC. "Update: multistate outbreak of mumps—United States, January 1--May 2, 2006." *MMWR* (May 26, 2006);55(20):559-63.

30. CDC. "Update: mumps outbreak—New York and New Jersey, June 2009-January 2010." *MMWR* (February 12, 2010).

31. Falco, M. "Mumps outbreak reaches nearly 2,000 in New York and New Jersey." *CNN* (February 12, 2010).

32. Mendelsohn, R. *How to Raise a Healthy Child...In Spite of Your Doctor.* (Ballantine Books, 1987):235.

33. CDC. "Mumps—United States, 1985-1988." *MMWR* 1989;38:101-105.

34. Savage, E., et al. "Mumps epidemic—United Kingdom, 2004-2005." *JAMA* (April 12, 2006);295(14):1636-37.

Rubella

What is rubella?

Rubella (or German Measles) is a contagious disease caused by a virus. Symptoms include a slight fever, rash, sore throat and runny nose. Lymph nodes on the back of the head, behind the ears, and on the side of the neck may become tender. In some instances, the joints become painful and swollen. Treatment mainly consists of allowing the disease to run its course. Medical intervention is seldom required. Symptoms usually disappear within a few days. Most cases confer permanent immunity; rubella rarely infects the same person twice.

Is rubella dangerous?

Rubella is usually a nonthreatening disease when contracted by children. The illness is ordinarily so mild it escapes detection or passes for a cold. However, if a pregnant woman develops rubella during the first trimester, her baby may be born with birth defects.

The rubella vaccine:

In 1969, the first live-virus rubella vaccine was licensed in the United States. Several European countries, Canada, and Japan also introduced rubella vaccines around this time. In 1979, a more potent live-virus rubella vaccine was sanctioned for use. Today, the current rubella vaccine is usually provided via MMR, but is available separately.

- Meruvax II—A preparation "of the Wistar Institute RA 27/3 strain of live attenuated rubella virus...adapted to and propagated in WI-38 human diploid lung fibroblasts" (fetal tissue). The growth medium is "supplemented with fetal bovine serum." This vaccine also contains sodium chloride, sodium phosphate, sucrose, sorbitol, hydrolyzed gelatin (an animal protein usually derived from cows or pigs), neomycin, and human serum albumin. Produced by Merck. Given in 2 doses.[1]

Safety

The drug company that produces the rubella vaccine publishes an extensive list of ailments known to have occurred following the rubella (or MMR) shot. These include arthritis, arthralgia, myalgia, encephalitis, Guillain-Barré syndrome, thrombocytopenia, leukocytosis, polyneuritis, polyneuropathy, optic neuritis, anaphylaxis, and death.[2] Numerous studies and frequent reports filed with the FDA's Vaccine Adverse Event Reporting System (VAERS) confirm these and other afflictions following rubella (or MMR) vaccination.

The rubella vaccine and ARTHRITIS:

As early as 1969—the same year that the rubella vaccine was initially licensed—the *New England Journal of Medicine* published a study documenting "arthritis after rubella vaccination."[3] The *American Journal of Diseases of Children* published another study showing that 10 percent of children developed joint problems following their rubella shots.[4] The *American Journal of Epidemiology* showed that 25 percent of women in their 20s, and 50 percent of women aged 25 to 33, had adverse joint symptoms following rubella vaccination.[5]

The *Journal of the American Medical Association* published data showing that 46 percent of women above 25 years of age developed acute arthritis following rubella vaccination.[6] The *American Journal of Epidemiology* published another study documenting "joint reactions in children vaccinated against rubella."[7] The *Journal of Pediatrics* also reported on several cases of "recurrent joint symptoms" in babies starting 2 to 7 weeks following their rubella vaccinations.[8]

The Lancet reported that chronic arthritis persisted for up to seven years in several women following their rubella shots.[9] The *Journal of Infectious Diseases* also recorded cases of chronic arthritis in women vaccinated against rubella.[10] A study published in *Annals of the Rheumatic Diseases* showed that 55 percent of women vaccinated against rubella developed arthritis or joint pain within four weeks.[11]

In 1991, the U.S. Vaccine Safety Committee acknowledged that the rubella vaccine causes both acute and long-term arthritis.[12] *Clinical Infectious Diseases* published a study documenting cases of "chronic arthritis" after rubella vaccination.[13] The *British Medical Journal* also showed that the rubella component of the MMR vaccine "is associated with an increased risk of episodes of joint and limb symptoms."[14] In 1998, the *Journal of Infectious Diseases* published yet another paper on "rubella vaccine-induced joint manifestations."[15]

Although many parents are unaware that the rubella (or MMR) vaccine can cause debilitating joint pain in their children, some make the connection. For example, one mother wrote the following:

"My baby daughter has been extremely ill for three weeks following her 12-month MMR shot. She had fever up to 102 degrees, vomiting, diarrhea, complete loss of appetite, and pain in her joints (knees, ankles, elbows and wrists). She has been learning American Sign Language, and began signing 'hurt' and pointing to her joints. It has been heartbreaking to see her lose the ability to stand and walk. I took a perfectly healthy, happy little girl to the doctor and our lives have been a nightmare. I will definitely trust my instincts and not take another chance, even though our pediatric office denies treatment if children are not up-to-date on their shots."[16]

—Concerned mother of a rubella (MMR)-vaccinated child

Another mother describes a similar experience:

"My daughter had a reaction to her MMR vaccine when she was 12 months old. Between 5 and 7 days after, she had high-pitched screaming that would last for 2 to 3 hours at a time. After taking her to the hospital, they found nothing wrong. She has had ankle pains ever since, for three years. She gets her 'ankle medicine' nearly every night."[17]

—Concerned mother of a rubella (MMR)-vaccinated child

Can the rubella vaccine cause BLOOD and NERVE DISORDERS?

The *New York State Journal of Medicine* published data on thrombocytopenia (a serious blood disorder) associated with rubella vaccination.[18] A study published in the *American Journal of Diseases of Children* documented neurological disorders following rubella shots. With one strain of the vaccine virus, researchers found "polyneuropathies" occurred at a rate of 2.2 cases per 1000 doses. Symptoms persisted for more than 2½ years in several children.[19]

The rubella vaccine and DIABETES:

Scientists have known for more than 30 years that "viral infection may play a part in the etiology of diabetes mellitus."[20] In fact, the rubella virus "consistently produces diabetes in man."[21] This is especially significant because if the wild rubella virus can cause illness, so can the manufactured rubella virus in the vaccine. In 1997, Dr. Harris Coulter testified before Congress on the link between vaccinations and juvenile-onset diabetes:

"Of the three vaccines making up the MMR shot, the rubella component is the major suspect because rubella itself, like mumps, is known to be a cause of diabetes, and the action of the vaccine resembles that of the disease. If the disease can cause diabetes, so can the vaccine."[22]

—Dr. Harris Coulter, medical historian

Additional research has shown that diabetes can be induced in laboratory animals by infecting them with the rubella virus. Authors of this study consider the most probable cause an immunological reaction—the formation of an autoimmune state in which the body becomes allergic to itself.[23] Scientists have also infected human pancreatic islet cells with rubella virus and noted "significant reductions in levels of secreted insulin."[24] Low insulin levels are associated with diabetes. Today, after more than 40 years of mass vaccinations with MMR, diabetes is an epidemic disease.

The rubella vaccine and CHRONIC FATIGUE SYNDROME:
Scientific studies have linked the new rubella vaccine introduced in 1979 to chronic fatigue syndrome, a debilitating immune system disorder. For example, *Medical Hypotheses* published research showing that although patients with chronic fatigue syndromes have elevated IgG serum antibodies to multiple common viruses, "only IgG *rubella* antibodies are positively correlated with the intensity of symptoms."[25] According to the author of the study, "In countries that routinely immunize children with the new [rubella] vaccine, adults might be persistently reexposed to the more provocative antigens of the new vaccine due to respiratory secretions..."[26] In other words, the rubella virus lingers in recently vaccinated children and can be spread to hypersensitive adults. *Clinical Ecology* published another study confirming that the vaccine strain of the rubella virus was a causative agent in the development of chronic fatigue syndrome.[27]

Efficacy

Prior to the introduction of the rubella vaccine in 1969, thousands of cases of rubella circulated throughout society. Most children contracted the disease and developed permanent protection. Thus, about 85 percent of the adult population was naturally immune; just 15 percent were susceptible to the disease.[28] After the vaccine was introduced, researchers noticed that cases of rubella were occurring in vaccinated populations. More than 10 years after a national immunization campaign with the rubella vaccine was instituted, *Pediatrics* published data indicating that about 15 percent of children in a well-vaccinated community remained susceptible to rubella. Serological analyses confirmed that about 15 percent of the adult population, including women of childbearing age, were still not protected from the disease—the same percentage as before vaccinations.[29-31]

The *Journal of the America Medical Association* published data showing that antibody levels after rubella vaccinations fell to half their high point within four years.[32] More data confirmed that many people vaccinated against rubella had no evidence of immunity within a few years. For example, Dr. Stanley Plotkin, Professor of Pediatrics at the University of Pennsylvania School of Medicine, showed that 36 percent of adolescent females who had been vaccinated against rubella lacked serological proof of immunity.[33]

According to the rubella vaccine manufacturer, a single injection of the vaccine has been shown to induce rubella-inhibiting antibodies in 97% of susceptible persons.[34] However, the *Journal of Infectious Diseases* published data showing that several people vaccinated against rubella and who later caught the disease—due to vaccine failures—had abundant antibodies to the rubella virus. Thus, antibody levels are not good indicators of immunity.[35] The manufacturer also claims that the rubella vaccine has "a high degree of protective efficacy."[36] However, this imprecise assessment is based upon a study done in 1972 on 18 vaccinated children. The vaccine failed in two of these children (11 percent) after just two years.[37]

What is the goal of rubella vaccination?

Mass rubella vaccination campaigns were never intended to protect vaccine recipients; the disease is usually harmless in children. Instead, the goal has always been to protect fetuses of rubella-susceptible pregnant women. As Dr. James Cherry, Professor of Pediatrics at UCLA, noted...

"The point of rubella immunization is not prevention of rubella but prevention of the congenital rubella syndrome."[38]
—James Cherry, MD, professor of pediatrics

Therefore, the vaccine's capacity to reduce the number of rubella cases is not nearly as significant as it's ability (or lack thereof) to protect fetuses from rubella-related birth defects.

Are rubella vaccine policies sensible?

Vaccine policymakers in the U.S. today recommend one dose of the rubella vaccine (via MMR) at 12 to 15 months of age plus a booster shot at 4 to 6 years. However, some authorities question whether children should be targeted for rubella vaccination.[39] Is it ethical for one herd —children—to be force-inoculated, denied natural immunity, and subjected to all of the potential side effects of the vaccine, so that another herd —pregnant women—may be theoretically protected?[40] Also, if the vaccine only offers temporary immunity, as studies indicate, and wears off in a few years, females vaccinated as children may actually have greater likelihoods of contracting rubella during their childbearing years.[41,42] On the other hand, if all children are given the opportunity to achieve natural immunity, by the time girls reach childbearing age about 85 percent will be naturally protected. Then, susceptible females—the one true, small group at risk—can be targeted for vaccination.[43,44]

The rubella vaccine shifted the disease to older age groups:
Vaccine strategies have altered the disease landscape. Dr. James Cherry noted that rubella vaccinations shifted age groups susceptible to the ailment:

"Essentially, we have controlled the disease in persons 14 years of age or younger but have given it a free hand in those 15 or older."[45]
—James Cherry, MD, professor of pediatrics

From 1966 to 1968, *before* the rubella vaccine was licensed, 77 percent of all cases occurred in persons 14 years of age or younger; just 23 percent occurred in persons 15 years of age or older.[46] By 1990, 81 percent of all rubella cases occurred in this older age group, with the greatest increases in persons 15 to 29 years old—*the prime childbearing years!*[47] By 1997, 85 percent of all rubella cases occurred in persons 15 years or older.[48]

Congenital rubella syndrome (CRS):
In 1941, Sir Norman Gregg, an Australian ophthalmologist, noticed that some women who caught rubella early in pregnancy gave birth to babies with disabilities, such as eye defects, hearing loss, heart disease, and learning problems.[49] Although some defects are short-lived or correctable, others are permanent.[50] However, not all pregnant women exposed to the virus give birth to injured babies.[51,52] Congenital rubella syndrome (CRS) occurs in less than 25 percent of infants born to women who contract rubella during the first trimester of pregnancy.[53] The risk of a single congenital defect declines to about 15 percent by the 16th week of pregnancy.[54] Defects are rare when the maternal infection occurs after the 20th week of gestation.[55]

Since 1969, when the rubella vaccine was introduced, the number of rubella cases has steadily declined. For example, in 1970 more than 56,000 cases were recorded in the U.S.; 3,904 in 1980; 1,125 in 1990; just 152 in 2000.[56,57] Authorities use this as evidence of the vaccine's efficacy and benefit to society. However, as noted earlier, the vaccine's capacity to reduce the number of rubella cases is inconsequential if it is unable to protect the unborn child from birth defects.[58]

In 1966, the year the government began keeping statistics on congenital rubella syndrome, there were 11 cases reported in the United States. In 1967, there were just 10 cases, with 14 more reported the following year. However, in 1969 the rubella vaccine was introduced and the CDC recorded 31 cases of CRS. In 1970, CRS cases skyrocketed to 77—a greater than 600 percent increase over pre-vaccine numbers. In 1971, there were another 68 cases. These figures remained high in later years.[59] (Although the U.S. government did not begin keeping official statistics on rubella and congenital rubella syndrome until 1966—when the CDC recorded 46,925 cases of rubella and 11 cases of CRS—some authorities assert that in 1964 and 1965 a rubella epidemic in the United States caused an *estimated* 12 million cases of rubella that resulted in "thousands of infections in pregnant women" and perhaps 20,000 cases of CRS. Estimates on the number of children who were born with some degree of deafness or blindness ranged from a low of 739 cases to a high of 10,000.)[60,61]

How do abortions influence CRS rates?

Some doctors recommend abortions to non-immune pregnant women when they are exposed to the rubella virus. James Cherry addressed this issue when he noticed that cases of CRS were declining even though the number of rubella infections in women of childbearing age remained stable.[62] Another researcher, Dr. Jean Joncas, also addressed this issue by noting that "the number of therapeutic abortions performed" when rubella is confirmed in pregnant women is rarely considered in evaluating decreases in the incidence of CRS.[63]

What do doctors think about the rubella vaccine?

The *New England Journal of Medicine* reported that one-third of all hospital employees rejected rubella shots; 81 percent of the doctors refused the vaccine, with senior staff physicians having an even lower participation rate.[64] The *Journal of the American Medical Association* reported similar figures: 78 percent of the doctors at the University of Southern California Medical Center would not comply with a rubella vaccination campaign, while 91 percent of the obstetricians and gynecologists (who work daily with pregnant women) refused to participate.[65,66]

When the doctors were questioned about their refusals, they confessed to being concerned about adverse reactions and did not think rubella vaccination was a priority. Even when these doctors were confronted with information that the potential for an outbreak existed, that the vaccine was safe, and that a history of previous rubella infection was an unreliable predictor of immunity, they still could not be persuaded to be vaccinated nor to endorse a rubella vaccination program. According to proponents of the vaccine, "Such reluctance on the part of physicians—especially influential, senior physicians—presents a formidable obstacle to convincing nonphysicians that such a program is safe, useful, and necessary."[67] This prompted Dr. Robert Mendelsohn to pose an ethical question:

"If doctors themselves are afraid of the [rubella] vaccine, why on earth should the law require that you and other parents allow them to administer it to your kids?"[68]
—Robert Mendelsohn, MD, pediatrician

Notes

1. Merck & Co., Inc. "Meruvax® (Rubella Virus Vaccine Live) Wistar RA 27/3 Strain." Product insert from the vaccine manufacturer (February 2006).

2. Ibid.

3. Gold, JA. "Arthritis after rubella vaccination of women." *New England Journal of Medicine* (July 10, 1969);281(2):109.

4. Spruance, SL., et al. "Joint complications associated with derivatives of HPV-77 rubella virus vaccine." *Amer J of Diseases of Children* 1971;122:105-111.

5. Swartz, TA., et al. "Clinical manifestations, according to age, among females given HPV-77 duck rubella vaccine." *American J of Epidemiology* 1971; 94:246-51.

6. Weibel, RE., et al. "Influence of age on clinical response to HPV-77 duck rubella vaccine." *Journal of the American Medical Association* 1972;222:805-807.

7. Austin, SM., et al. "Joint reactions in children vaccinated against rubella. I. Comparison of two vaccines. *Amer J of Epidemiology* (Jan. 1972);95(1):53-58.

8. Spruance, SL., et al. "Recurrent joint symptoms in children vaccinated with HPV-77DK12 rubella vaccine." *Journal of Pediatrics* 1972;80(3):413-17.

9. Tingle, AJ., et al. "Prolonged arthritis, viraemia, hypogammaglobulinaemia, and failed seroconversion following rubella immunisation." *Lancet* 1984;1:1475-76.

10. Tingle, AJ., et al. "Postpartum rubella immunization: association with development of prolonged arthritis, neurological sequelae, and chronic rubella viremia." *Journal of Infectious Diseases* 1985;152:606-612.

11. Tingle, AJ., et al. "Rubella-associated arthritis. Comparative study of joint manifestations associated with natural rubella infection and RA 27/3 rubella immunisation." *Annals of the Rheumatic Diseases* 1986; 45:110-114.

12. Institute of Medicine. *Adverse Effects of Pertussis and Rubella Vaccines.* (Washington, DC: Natl Acad Press, 1991).

13. Howson, CP., et al. "Chronic arthritis after rubella vaccination." *Clin Infect Dis,* (Aug 1992);15(2):307-312.

14. Benjamin, CM., et al. "Joint and limb symptoms in children after immunisation with measles, mumps, and rubella vaccine." *British Medical J* 1992;304:1075-78.

15. Mitchell, LA., et al. "HLA-DR class II associations with rubella vaccine-induced joint manifestations." *J Infect Dis* (January 1998);177(1):5-12.

16. Thinktwice Global Vaccine Institute. Unsolicited case reports submitted by concerned parents. www.thinktwice.com

17. Ibid.

18. Bartos, HR. "Thrombocytopenia associated with rubella vaccination." *NY State J Med* (February 15, 1972);72(4):499.

19. Schaffner, W., et al. "Polyneuropathy following rubella immunization: a follow-up study & review of the problem." *Amer. J. of Diseases of Children* 1974;127:684-688.

20. Menser, M., et al. "Rubella infection and diabetes mellitus." *The Lancet* (January 14, 1978):57-60.

21. Ibid.

22. Coulter, Harris. "Childhood vaccinations and Juvenile-Onset (Type-1) diabetes." Congressional Testimony. *Committee on Appropriations, Subcommittee on Labor, Health and Human Services...* (April 16, 1997).

23. Rayfield, EJ., et al. "Rubella virus-induced diabetes in the hamster." *Diabetes* (December 1986);35:1278-1281.

24. Numazaki, K., et al. "Infection of cultured human fetal pancreatic islet cells by rubella virus." *American Journal of Clinical Pathology* 1989;91:446-451.

25. Allen, AD. "Is RA27/3 rubella immunization a cause of chronic fatigue?" *Medical Hypotheses* 1988; 27:217-220.

26. Ibid.

27. Lieberman, AD. "The role of the rubella virus in the chronic fatigue syndrome." *Clinical Ecology* 1991; 7(3):51-54.

28. Cherry, JD. "The 'new' epidemiology of measles and rubella." *Hospital Practice* (July 1980):56.

29. Lawless, M., et al. "Rubella susceptibility in sixth-graders." *Pediatrics* (June 1980);65:1086-1089.

30. Bart, KJ., et al. "Universal immunization to interrupt rubella." *Review of Infectious Diseases* 1985;7(1):S177-84.

31. Crowder, M., et al. "Rubella susceptibility in young women of rural East Texas: 1980 and 1985." *Texas Med* 1987;83:43-47.

32. Herrmann, KL., et al. "Rubella antibody persistence after immunization." *JAMA* 1982;247(2):193-196.

33. Mendelsohn, R. *But Doctor, About That Shot...The Risks of Immunizations and How to Avoid Them* (Evanston, IL: The People's Doctor Newsletter, 1988):31.

34. See Note 1.

35. Tingle, AJ., et al. "Failed rubella immunization in adults: association with immunologic and virological abnormalities." *Journal of Infectious Diseases* 1985; 151(2):330-336.

36. See Note 1.

37. Leibhaber, H., et al. "Vaccination with RA 27/3 rubella vaccine." *Am. J. Dis. Child* (February 1972):133-136.

38. See Note 28, p. 55.

39. Schoenbaum, SC., et al. "Epidemiology of congenital rubella syndrome: the role of maternal parity." *J of the American Medical Assoc* 1975;233:151-155.

40. Diodati, C. *Immunization: History, Ethics, Law and Health.* (Windsor, Ontario, Canada: Integral Aspects Inc., 1999):17-19.

41. WHO Copenhagen. "Expanded programme on immunization—report of the meeting of national programme managers," 1989.

42. See Note 33, p. 239-240.

43. Ibid.

44. Spika, JS., et al. "Rubella vaccination: a course becomes clear." *Canadian Med Assoc J* (July 15, 1983);129(2):106-110.

45. See Note 28, p. 55.

46. CDC. "Rubella and congenital rubella syndrome—United States, 1985-1988. *MMWR* 1989;38:173-178.

47. CDC. "Current trends increase in rubella and congenital rubella syndrome—United States, 1988-1990." *MMWR Weekly* (Feb 15, 1991);40(6):93-99.

48. Baker, B. "Rubella ready for possible worldwide eradication." *Pediatric News* 2000;34(1):18.

49. Meissner, HC., et al. "Elimination of rubella from the United States: a milestone on the road to global elimination." *Pediatrics* (Mar 2006);117(3):933-35.

50. "Rubella—Public Health Information Sheet." *March of Dimes Birth Defects Foundation* (White Plains, NY: October 1984). Extracted from CDC data.

51. Victorian Government Health Information. "Rubella (German measles)." *State Government of Victoria, Australia, Human Services*. www.health.vic.gov.au

52. See Note 47.

53. See Note 51.

54. Ibid.

55. Ibid.

56. CDC. "Summary of notifiable diseases, United States, 1995." *MMWR Weekly* (October 25, 1996);44(53):1-87.

57. CDC. "Notifiable diseases/deaths in selected cities weekly information." *MMWR Weekly* (Jan 5, 2001);49(51):1167-1174.

58. See Note 28, p. 55.

59. See Note 56.

60. Meissner, HC., et al. "Elimination of rubella from the United States: a milestone on the road to global elimination." *Pediatrics* 2006; Vol. 117(3):933-935.

61. Lockett, et al. "Deaf-blind children with maternal rubella: implications for adult services." *American Annals of the Deaf* 1980, Vol. 125(8).

62. See Note 28, p.55.

63. Joncas, J. "Preventing the congenital rubella syndrome by vaccinating women at risk." *Canadian Medical Association Journal* (July 15, 1983);129(2):110-112.

64. Polk, BF., et al. "An outbreak of rubella among hospital personnel." *New England J of Medicine* 1980;303:541-545.

65. Orenstein, WA., et al. "Rubella vaccine and susceptible hospital employees: poor physician participation." *JAMA* (February 20, 1981);245(7):711-713.

66. Sacks, JJ., et al. "Employee rubella screening program." *Journal of the American Medical Association* 1983;249:2675-2678.

67. Preblud, SR., et al. "Rubella vaccination of hospital employees (editorial)." *Journal of the American Medical Association* (February 20, 1981);245(7):737.

68. See Note 33, p. 241.

MMR

What is MMR?

MMR is an abbreviation for measles, mumps, and rubella—three common childhood illnesses up until the mid-1970s. Vaccines are available for each of these diseases. However, in the 1980s they were combined into a single "three-in-one" MMR shot.

The MMR vaccine:

- MMR II—A compound preparation made by mixing three separate live-virus vaccines into a single shot: Attenuvax (for measles), Mumpsvax (for mumps), and Meruvax II (for rubella). Contains attenuated live measles and mumps viruses propagated in chick embryo cell culture, plus "the Wistar RA 27/3 strain of live attenuated rubella virus propagated in WI-38 human diploid lung fibroblasts" (cultured from an aborted human fetus). In addition, the growth medium for the three live viruses is a buffered salt solution "supplemented with fetal bovine serum." Each dose also includes sodium chloride, sodium phosphate, sucrose, sorbitol, hydrolyzed gelatin, glutamate, neomycin, and human albumin. Produced by Merck. Given in 2 doses.[1]
- ProQuad—A compound preparation made by mixing four separate live-virus vaccines into a single shot: Attenuvax, Mumpsvax, Meruvax II, and Varivax (for chickenpox).

Safety

The drug company that makes the MMR vaccine publishes an extensive list of warnings, contraindications, and adverse reactions associated with this triple shot. These may be found in the vaccine package insert (available from any doctor giving MMR) and in the *Physician's Desk Reference* (PDR) at the library. Afflictions affecting blood, lymphatic, digestive, cardiovascular, immune, nervous, respiratory, and sensory systems have been reported after MMR. (For specific ailments linked to MMR, read the safety sections in the chapters on measles, mumps, and rubella.)

The case reports on the following page were taken directly from the FDA's Vaccine Adverse Event Reporting System (VAERS).[2] They are just a small sample of the potential side effects that are possible when babies receive the MMR vaccine. (Case numbers precede report summaries.)

MMR Vaccine: VAERS Case Reports

▶71322: A one-year-old female developed seizures and bacterial meningitis two days after receiving MMR. She required extended hospitalization.

▶35283: A 14-month-old boy received the MMR vaccine and within 24 hours suffered a brain injury and respiratory arrest.

▶36455: A 14-month-old boy developed apnea, brain edema, cardiac arrest, diabetic ketoacidosis, and subarachnoid hemorrhage two days after receiving MMR. He died three days later.

▶75202: A 15-month-old boy received MMR and four days later became blind, developed convulsions, encephalopathy, and movement disorder. He spent four months in the hospital.

▶34373: A 15-month-old boy developed a rash on his body three days after receiving MMR, became flaccid, was rushed to the hospital and died.

▶39041: A 15-month-old girl received the MMR vaccine, developed a fever and died the following day.

▶50505: A 16-month-old female received the MMR vaccine and "began drinking and urinating excessively" eight days later. Her blood sugar levels were tested and she was diagnosed with diabetes.

▶43310: A 17-month-old female received the MMR vaccine and within one day developed symptoms leading to ataxia, abnormal coordination, and leukoencephalopathy, She was hospitalized.

▶55312: A 17-month-old boy developed unsafe blood platelet levels and thrombocytopenia the same day he received MMR. He was hospitalized.

▶75498: A 17-month-old girl developed anemia, bone marrow depression, encephalitis, leukopenia, mouth sores, thrombocytopenia, and visual disturbances eleven days after receiving MMR. Extended hospitalization was required.

▶41319: An 18-month-old boy received the MMR vaccine and 13 days later began seizuring, stopped breathing and went into cardiac arrest. He was hospitalized for 14 days.

▶54616: A 19-month-old baby developed grand mal convulsions and respiratory arrest nine days after receiving MMR. He was airlifted to a children's hospital; en route he had 10 more grand mal seizures and went into full cardiac arrest.

▶101589: A 19-month-old female received MMR and nine days later died. According to the autopsy, "Apart from being too old, the patient fulfills all criteria for sudden infant death syndrome (SIDS)."

▶51544: A 20-month-old baby received MMR, stopped eating and died the following day.

▶44783: A 2-year-old boy suffered an allergic asthmatic reaction five hours after receiving MMR vaccine. According to the official report, he "would have died if someone else had not been in the room" at the time.

▶35087: A 2-year-old girl received the MMR vaccine and ten days later developed 2-3 inch diameter bruises on her trunk, arms and legs. Her blood platelet count dropped to unsafe levels consistent with thrombocytopenia and she was hospitalized.

Case Reports by Parents

▸ *"My 12-year-old had a seizure within 10 minutes of his second MMR. His head rolled side to side and his arms jerked a couple of times. He was unaware of this, so he must have blanked out."*

▸ *"My daughter had a serious reaction to MMR at 22 months. She developed brain damage after a fever of 106 degrees. She also has seizures which are unresponsive to medication, damage to the nerves of her eyes, and learning disabilities that she battles every day. We took her case to court and lost. The doctor who testified on their behalf stated that the government only called him in when they wanted a finding in their favor. What a setup! Of course they don't have to live with the frustrations and expense of raising these vaccine-damaged children."*

▸ *"When my daughter was two years old, she received her MMR shot. Five days later, she had a high fever and seizures. Now she has a hearing loss."*

▸ *"My daughter received her second MMR when she was three years old. Shortly after, she started having a problem with her hearing."*

▸ *"My son recently contracted SSPE, a measles-virus illness. It all started three years ago when his health deteriorated to where he could not function—no walking, talking or head movement whatsoever. My son never had measles but he had the MMR vaccination. The gestation period for SSPE is from 2 to 12 years. It doesn't take a brain surgeon to figure out what caused my son's ailment, but trying to prove it is a different matter."*

▸ *"My once healthy son developed urticaria eight days after his MMR. Then he developed epileptic seizures. Years later, the seizures really took hold and, to cut this long and tragic story short, he underwent emergency brain surgery. (The measles vaccine virus was found in his brain.) After that he was a changed youngster, his personality was lost, and he behaved in a basic, instinctive way."*[3]

Efficacy

Prior to the introduction of the measles, mumps and rubella vaccines, thousands of cases of measles, mumps and rubella occurred every year. Today, these numbers are greatly reduced. However, unlike the natural diseases, the MMR vaccine does not confer permanent immunity. The medical literature contains many examples of MMR failures. Thus, people who receive MMR may still be susceptible to the three diseases.

MMR and AUTISM

Many parents report that their perfectly healthy children became autistic after receiving the MMR vaccine. (Autism is a complex autoimmune and developmental disability. Common symptoms include inadequate verbal and social skills, repetitive behavior patterns, little or no interest in human contact, self-destructive behavior, and gastrointestinal anomalies.) The affected children were developing normally, then regressed after receiving the triple-virus shot, losing their previously acquired skills. Most medical authorities deny a connection between the MMR vaccine and autism. However, Dr. Andrew Wakefield investigated previously normal children who subsequently suffered from intestinal abnormalities and regressive developmental disorder, including a loss of acquired skills. In many cases, "onset of symptoms was after measles, mumps, and rubella immunization."[4] Further research uncovered a possible explanation:

Atypical patterns of exposure to common childhood infections—measles, mumps, rubella and chickenpox—have been associated with autism and autistic regression.... A close temporal relationship in the exposure to two of these infections during periods of susceptibility may compound both the risk and severity of autism.... Although historically these rare patterns of exposure may have accounted for only a small proportion of autism, the widespread use of a combination of the candidate agents in a single vaccine [MMR] may have changed this.[5]

In other words, a young child exposed to one viral disease (measles, mumps, rubella, or chickenpox) usually recovers. If the child is exposed to another viral disease weeks or months later, once again, recovery is expected. However, a young child exposed to two or more viral diseases at the same time is at increased risk for adverse complications. The MMR vaccine contains three viruses. Children vaccinated with MMR are exposed to three viral diseases at the same time.

An earlier study published in the *American Journal of Epidemiology* identified in utero and infant exposures as periods of apparent susceptibility, when both the brain and immune system are undergoing rapid development.[6] Thus, fetuses and young children are especially prone to adverse consequences if they contract two or more viral infections concurrently.

Wakefield elaborated on the increased perils of being exposed to more than one virus at a time:

One important pattern of infection that may increase the risk of delayed disease is where different viruses interact, either with each other or both interact with the host immune system simultaneously. Virologic data support the possibility of a compound effect of multiple concurrent viral exposures influencing...the risk of autism.[7]

Is it safer to receive MMR as three separate shots?

Dr. Wakefield theorized that if a child who is exposed to two or more *wild* viral infections around the same time is at increased risk for autism, then a child who is injected with three live viruses via the MMR vaccine may also be at risk, if not more so. Thus, Wakefield proposed separating the measles, mumps and rubella vaccines from the three-in-one MMR shot—the way they were in the 1970s prior to being combined—and giving them individually over the course of several weeks or months. His solution would satisfy immunization recommendations designed to protect against the three diseases while safeguarding against the risk of autism:

If, following thorough independent scientific investigation, it emerges that autistic...disorders are causally related to a compound influence of the component viruses of MMR, whether these viruses have been encountered naturally or in the vaccine, then through judicious use of the vaccines, one may have a means for preventing the disease [autism]. Spacing the single vaccines, thereby dissociating the exposures that, together, may constitute the risk, provides a way of not only preventing the acute measles, mumps and rubella infections, but also, potentially, the risk of one of the most devastating diseases that it has been our misfortune to encounter.[8]

For families choosing to vaccinate their children, Wakefield's proposal to separate the shots seems like a prudent approach, especially since recipients of MMR are injected with three unique viruses—plus other questionable ingredients—all at once. Moreover, the scientific literature contains ample documentation linking MMR to serious adverse reactions. Thus, when Wakefield's research was first publicized, concerned parents rejected MMR and demanded instead the individual shots. Some doctors initially supported Wakefield's suggestion and complied with parents' requests. However, *the individual measles, mumps and rubella vaccines may cause severe adverse reactions* as well. These are listed by the vaccine manufacturer and documented in numerous studies.

MMR was initially administered as three separate shots (during the 1960s and 1970s), rarely at the same time. Thus, early reports of adverse reactions could be attributed to a particular vaccine. Later, when the three-in-one MMR shot replaced the individual vaccines it became much more difficult to link a bad reaction to either the measles, mumps, or rubella portions of the shot. Today, MMR is often given in combination with other vaccines as well, making it even more difficult to determine if one vaccine caused an adverse reaction, or if all of the vaccines given at once overwhelmed the recipient's immune system. (For more information about this topic, read the chapter on multiple vaccines given simultaneously.)

Note: In January 2010, a British medical panel concluded that Dr. Wakefield had violated ethics rules, prompting *The Lancet* to retract his 1998 research paper which suggested that MMR may be linked to autism.[9] However, according to Wakefield, "the allegations against me and my colleagues are both unfounded and unjust and I invite anyone to examine the contents of these proceedings and come to their own conclusion."[10]

Why are the three vaccines combined?

The three vaccines—measles, mumps and rubella—are combined into a single shot for *convenience,* not safety or efficacy. In fact, when 180 Swiss physicians analyzed 320 scientific works from around the world they concluded that *there is no medical foundation for combining measles, mumps and rubella into a single shot.* Speaking as a group, these doctors formally rejected a compulsory MMR immunization campaign:

> *One thing is...unmistakably clear from the example of the USA: the MMR immunization campaign...has elements of compulsion that work into the sphere of individual rights. Since the USA has enforced a 95 percent immunization level by means of obligatory vaccination, unexpected epidemics now make rigorous, police-enforced measures necessary, with quarantines, exclusions from school, and house-to-house vaccinations.*
>
> *These three childhood diseases necessitate the fulfillment of three completely different objectives to which it is impossible to do justice with a single combined injection.... After a careful analysis of the relevant material [we, the 180 unified physicians] reject the state MMR campaign... [and] advocate a very restrained, individually adjusted immunization practice which takes account of the different nature of the problems relating to the three childhood diseases, does not fundamentally alter the epidemiology of the three diseases, and respects parents' freedom of choice.[11]*

Can the three vaccines be administered separately?

Yes. The three vaccines—for measles, mumps and rubella—can be administered separately because they are manufactured individually as

MMR and AUTISM: Case Reports by Parents

▸ *"After my son's MMR at 12 months, his development and personality changed. He would stare off and not notice anything, even the waving of my hand in front of his face. His personality became nothing—he lost all words and still has none. It is hard to see my only son lose his personality and life to a shot."*

▸ *"My son received the MMR shot shortly after his first birthday. I complained to his doctor when he did not walk, talk or respond as a normal one-year-old. I was told that the shots would not have that reaction. He was diagnosed as mentally retarded, autistic, and Tourette's syndrome."*

▸ *"My son is vaccine-injured. After his 15-month vaccines, he could no longer stand, quit talking, and had terrible diarrhea that still isn't resolved six years later. He is autistic, and his spinal fluid contains vaccine-strain measles virus."*

▸ *"When our beautiful, healthy, only son was 15 months old, he was given MMR. In four days he was at death's door with meningitis. He could no longer speak, walk, eat, or see. His behavior could best be described as autistic."*

▸ *"My 10-year-old son was healthy until 9 days after his MMR. He had seizures and a measles rash, then lost his few words of speech over the next week."*

▸ *"My granddaughter was vaccinated for MMR. Ten days later, she stopped talking, standing, and developed a shakiness that affects her upper body."*

▸ *"I am the mother of an 8-year-old who was stricken with severe epilepsy and mild autism following his MMR shots when he was 18 months old. He has suffered more than 50 seizures, some requiring hospitalization."*

▸ *"My friend works for a lady who has 3 autistic children. The girl was 2 years old when she got her MMR; within 48 hours she could no longer function like a 2-year-old. She was later diagnosed with autism, the same for the boys."*

▸ *"My first child received MMR when I was pregnant, and exposed my unborn baby to the rubella virus. He was born deaf with ADHD and autistic traits."*

▸ *"When my son was a baby, I got him all of the required shots. He reacted badly to MMR and has been diagnosed with pervasive developmental disorder."*

▸ *"Exactly 14 days after my son's MMR, he had measles-type and mumps-type reactions. He is now autistic. He also has leaky gut syndrome and asthma. My son was in PERFECT health up until the day of his reaction. He lost all powers of speech on that day and has never regained them."*

▸ *"Prior to my son's MMR, he said loads of words. Now he has little speech and is autistic. If I could turn back the clock, I would, but I have to live with the fact that we did not protect him; we let them damage him beyond repair."*

▸ *"My grandson had his MMR and immediately showed signs that were puzzling to us. He stopped talking, only screamed, and started to walk on his toes. Doctors were no help. We were finally told he has 'autistic traits.'"*[12]

Attenuvax, Mumpsvax, and Meruvax II *before* they are mixed into a single MMR shot. (Details can be found in the separate chapters on measles, mumps and rubella.) However, health authorities in the United States, England and elsewhere have restricted or forbidden this option. Most doctors either cannot or will not provide parents with the individual shots. They claim that if these vaccines are administered separately over several weeks, rather than all at once, children will remain vulnerable to disease. One mother voices her concerns:

> *"I read that ultra-sensitive kids do better with individual components of MMR rather than the three-in-one shot. Our son has had sensory issues so we would like to have him vaccinated separately, but I can't find the individual vaccines and our doctor won't help."*[13]

Another parent voices similar concerns:

> *"How can we get MMR for our son in three separate doses instead of one MMR shot? Our health department says that it's impossible."*[14]

Notes

1. Merck & Co., Inc. "M-M-R®II (Measles, Mumps, and Rubella Virus Vaccine Live)." Product insert from the vaccine manufacturer (Issued: December 2007).

2. National Vaccine Information Center. "MedAlerts: access to the U.S. government's Vaccine Adverse Event Reporting System (VAERS)." www.medalerts.org

3. Thinktwice Global Vaccine Institute. Unsolicited case reports submitted by concerned parents. www.thinktwice.com

4. Wakefield, AJ., et al. "Ileal-lymphoid-nodular hyperplasia, non-specific colitis, and pervasive developmental disorder in children." *The Lancet* 1998; 351:637-641.

5. "Autism: Present Challenges, Future Needs—Why the Increased Rates?" *Government Reform Committee Hearing,* Washington, DC. (April 6, 2000.) As cited in Andrew Wakefield's testimony.

6. Deykin, EY., et al. "Viral exposure and autism." *Am J Epid* 1979;109:628-38.

7. See Note 5.

8. Ibid.

9. Harris, G. "Journal retracts 1998 paper linking autism to vaccines." *New York Times* (February 2, 2010). www.nytimes.com

10. Maugh II, TH. "Andrew Wakefield responds to article about journal retraction of autism study report." *LA Times* (February 3, 2010). www.latimesblogs.latimes.com

11. Albonico, H., Klein, P., et al. "The immunization campaign against measles, mumps and rubella—coercion leading to a realm of uncertainty: medical objections to a continued MMR immunization campaign in Switzerland." *Journal of Anthroposophical Medicine* (Spring1992);9(1).

12. See Note 3.

13. Ibid.

14. Ibid.

Autism

In 1943, the well-known child psychiatrist, Dr. Leo Kanner, announced his discovery of 11 cases of a new mental disorder. He noted that "the condition differs markedly and uniquely from anything reported so far..."[1] This condition soon became known as autism.

What is autism?

Autism (often referred to as autistic spectrum disorder, Asperger's syndrome, or pervasive developmental disorder) is a complex developmental disability that affects the brain, immune system and gastrointestinal tract. This condition usually appears during the first three years of life and often strikes after an early childhood of normal development. Mental and social regression are not uncommon. Although the severity of the affliction varies from child to child, the following symptoms are typical: inadequate verbal and social skills, impaired speech, repetition of words, bizarre or repetitive behavior patterns, uncontrollable head-banging, screaming fits, arm flapping, little or no interest in human contact, unresponsiveness to parents and other people, extreme resistance to minor changes in the home environment, self-destructive behavior, hypersensitivity to sensory stimuli, diarrhea, constipation, food allergies, and an inability to care for oneself.

How common is autism?

According to several researchers who investigated Kanner's claims, autism was extremely rare prior to 1943. Using Kanner's own case definition of autism, Dr. Darold Treffert calculated a rate of less than 1 in 10,000 during the 1950s.[2] In 1966, Dr. Victor Lotter found the rate to be 4.1 per 10,000 children.[3] However, by the 1980s over 4500 new cases were being reported every year in the United States alone.[4] In 1997, the CDC reported that 1 of every 500 children is autistic (20 per 10,000).[5] In 2007, the CDC showed that autism affects 1 of every 150 U.S. children (67 per 10,000).[6] Two years later, in October 2009, the CDC released new figures showing that autism affects 1 of every 91 children (110 per 10,000).[7] This figure is 1 in 58 for boys.[8] "We have an epidemic on our hands," exclaimed Congressman Christopher Smith.[9] Congressman Chip Pickering described the epidemic in more sobering terms:

"More children will be diagnosed with autism this year than AIDS, diabetes and cancer combined."[10]
—**Congressman Chip Pickering**

What causes autism?

When the first cases of autism began to appear in the 1940s, researchers were puzzled by the high incidence of autistic children being born into well-educated families. Over 90 percent of the parents were high school graduates. Nearly three-fourths of the fathers and one-half of the mothers had graduated from college. Many had professional careers. As a result, scientists unsuccessfully tried to link autism to genetic factors in upper class populations.[11] Meanwhile, psychiatrists, unaware of the neurological basis of the illness, sought psychological explanations. The mother was accused of not providing an emotionally secure home environment, and presumed to be the cause of her afflicted child's ailment.[12,13]

Today, researchers have discounted these earlier notions but still do not have a complete understanding of this condition. Although autism has been linked to biological and neurological differences in the brain, and genetic factors appear to play a role, no single cause has been identified. However, recent dramatic increases in the number of children stricken with this debilitating ailment—coincident with the introduction of new vaccines—may shed some light on this medical mystery.

Autism and compulsory vaccination programs:

The first cases of autism in the United States occurred shortly after the pertussis vaccine became available. When the pertussis vaccine was initially introduced (during the late 1930s), only rich and educated parents who sought the very best for their children, and who could afford a private doctor, were in a position to request the newest medical advancements. (Remember how researchers were puzzled by the high incidence of autistic children being born into well-educated and upper class families.) However, by the 1960s and 1970s parents all over the country, within every income and educational level, were seeking help for their autistic children. Socioeconomic disparities began to disappear during this period. Today, autism is evenly distributed among all social classes and ethnic groups.[14] Once again this puzzled researchers. Many simply concluded that earlier studies were flawed, but there is an explanation. Free vaccines at public health clinics didn't yet exist in the 1940s and 1950s. Compulsory vaccination programs were still on the horizon. However, as vaccine programs grew, parents from across the socioeconomic spectrum gained equal access to them. The growing number of children suffering from this new illness directly coincided with the increasing popularity of mandated vaccination programs during these same years. Autistic children were now being found within every kind of family in greater numbers than ever before imagined.[15]

In the 1980s and 1990s, cases of autism soared once again. For example, the California Department of Health examined the number of people with autism requiring developmental resources. There were increases each year from 1987 to 1998, with an overall increase of 273 percent during this period. Services for all other developmental disabilities increased by no more than 50 percent during this same period.[16] The U.S. Department of Education (DOE) showed even greater increases: from 1991 to 1997, the number of children with autism requiring special education services increased 556 percent.[17] Other countries have experienced similar increases. Impartial autism researchers do not attribute these increases to better diagnostic skills nor to expanded diagnostic categories. Several analysts implicate vaccines—especially the three-in-one live-virus MMR shot introduced and vigorously marketed during this period. Analysts also blame the busier vaccine schedule (read the chapter on multiple vaccines) and the greater number of mercury-containing vaccines mandated for children. In fact, each year as the number of required vaccines rise, autism cases soar. Aluminum-containing vaccines may also be a factor.

MMR and Autism

In 1996, Dr. Hugh Fudenberg, director of the *NeuroImmuno Therapeutics Research Foundation,* published a pilot study on infantile onset autism and noted that 75 percent of his subjects exhibited their initial symptoms within one week of vaccination.[18] Dr. Sudhir Gupta, world-renowned immunologist, also noted an association between the onset of autistic symptoms and vaccination, especially MMR. He presented his findings at the *National Autism Association* in Chicago.[19] Dr. Bernard Rimland, director of the internationally recognized *Autism Research Institute,* spoke at the Chicago conference as well. He confirmed that overzealous childhood vaccine programs are a leading cause of autism epidemics.[20]

The Yazbak autism studies:

In 1999, Dr. Edward Yazbak published two separate studies showing significant correlations between MMR and autism. In the first study, mothers who received an MMR vaccine prior to conception and again shortly after giving birth, increased their child's risk of autism when they breastfed their child *and* later permitted the child to receive an MMR shot.[21] In the second study, six of seven children (86%) born to mothers who received an MMR vaccine prior to conception and again during pregnancy were diagnosed with autism. The seventh child had developmental problems.[22]

In 2000, Dr. Yazbak published a third study demonstrating that "the administration of a live virus vaccine booster (MMR) to a mother around conception, pregnancy, or delivery" may result in a child with autism. In this study, 22 of 22 mothers (100%) who had received a live virus vaccine during this crucial period "had at least one child develop autism in connection with or following such a vaccination.... In many instances, the children's autistic manifestations reportedly started or worsened after they received their first MMR vaccine." Dr. Yazbak concluded that giving live virus vaccines (MMR or rubella) to a mother just before or during early pregnancy, or in the postpartum period, "may not be safe or wise.... The role of vaccines in precipitating autism should therefore become the focus of extensive and unbiased research."[23]

On April 23, 2001, the newly created Institute of Medicine (IOM) Immunization Review Committee, issued a report concluding that "the evidence favors rejection of the causal relationship at the population level between MMR vaccine and autistic spectrum disorders." However...

"The proposed biological models linking MMR vaccination to autism spectrum disorders, although far from established, are...not disproved."[24]
—Institute of Medicine Immunization Review Committee

Suppressed data:
On November 21, 2002, Congressman Dan Burton wrote to President Bush urging him to host a White House conference "to galvanize a national effort to determine why autism has reached epidemic proportions."[25] Four days later, attorneys for the U.S. government responded by asking a federal court to conceal important documents linking vaccines to autism. They argued that only the government has the right to decide what vaccine evidence can be released to the public. According to Jeff Kim, a lawyer representing hundreds of families whose children became autistic after receiving MMR, sealing important documents and creating "a shroud of secrecy" over them solely benefits vaccine manufacturers.[26] A few days later, the *New York Times* published a commentary by Stephen Gillers, a legal ethicist, providing clarity on this issue:

"When a court is asked to suppress information that might help vindicate legal claims, or that reveals a continuing public danger or unethical behavior by powerful people or institutions, secrecy is intolerable. The harm is made worse when a judge, a public official, is asked to use public power to inflict it."[27]
—Stephen Gillers, legal ethicist, New York Times

A warning cry:
In February 2006, Dr. Peter Fletcher, former Chief Scientific Officer at the U.K. Department of Health, and former Medical Assessor to the Committee on Safety of Medicines (responsible for deciding if vaccines are safe), publicly acknowledged that he has seen a "steady accumulation of evidence" from scientists worldwide that the MMR vaccine is causing brain damage in some children. Dr. Fletcher elaborated:

"There are very powerful people in positions of great authority in Britain and elsewhere who have staked their reputations and careers on the safety of MMR, and they are willing to do almost anything to protect themselves.... It's entirely possible that the immune systems of a small minority simply cannot cope with the challenge of the three live viruses in the MMR jab and the ever-increasing vaccine load in general.... The refusal by governments to evaluate [MMR] risks properly will make this one of the greatest scandals in medical history."[28]
—**Dr. Peter Fletcher, Chief Scientist, Dept. of Health, UK**

Mercury in Vaccines: A Link to Autism

In 1929, Eli Lilly, a vaccine manufacturer, developed and registered thimerosal under the trade name Merthiolate.[29] Thimerosal is nearly 50 percent mercury by weight.[30] Mercury is the most toxic element on earth, after plutonium. Even very low amounts—whether inhaled, eaten, or placed on the skin—can cause nervous system and brain damage.[31] In the 1930s and 1940s, thimerosal was added to pertussis vaccines (and DPT) as an anti-bacterial preservative.[32] In the 1990s, additional mercury-laced vaccines were added to the mandatory schedule of childhood shots. Starting in 1991, infants received several doses of the mercury-filled hepatitis B vaccine, with the first shot given just hours after birth. Multiple doses of the mercury-filled Hib vaccine were given to babies as well.

Throughout the infamous era of mercury-tainted vaccines—sadly, still occurring—outraged parents of vaccine-damaged children pleaded with anyone who would listen: Why is mercury being injected into our precious babies? No one had an answer. In fact, the medical community refused to even acknowledge their pleas—despite a secret memo from 1991. Apparently, pharmaceutical executives had calculated that 6-month-old babies who received their recommended shots could receive a mercury dose up to 87 times higher than federal guidelines for the maximum daily consumption of mercury from fish![33] Eight years later, health officials finally recommended removing thimerosal from vaccines.

In July 1999, health officials recommended that vaccine manufacturers eliminate thimerosal as a preservative "as soon as possible."[34] However, newly released documents show that the CDC was simultaneously working behind the scenes to discourage thimerosal's removal. For example, when a major vaccine manufacturer—SmithKline Beecham—contacted the CDC shortly after its announcement, and offered to immediately begin supplying mercury-free DTaP vaccines for children, the CDC rejected the offer.[35,36] Perhaps a sharp plunge in autism rates would seem too obvious. One federal health official declared...

"If CDC were basing its decision on safety alone, it would have taken SmithKline up on its offer. That's a no-brainer, so there were other considerations. Immediate withdrawal would send a strong message: 'We messed up!' I don't think they wanted to send that message to parents, the public, or those considering legal action."[37]
—**Federal health official**

The CDC was also concerned that "an immediate withdrawal might discredit international vaccine programs."[38] The World Health Organization (WHO) has urged the CDC against banning thimerosal in U.S. vaccines because it might elicit objections to immunization programs overseas. WHO is now injecting children in developing countries with the same amount of mercury that U.S. children received at their highest exposures, but in less time.[39] According to Dr. John Clements, WHO vaccine advisor...

"My mandate...is to make sure...that 100 million are immunized...this year, next year and for many years to come, and that will have to be with thimerosal-containing vaccines."[40]
—**Dr. John Clements, WHO vaccine advisor**

The Simpsonwood Gathering:
In June 2000, a top-secret meeting of health officials and government scientists occurred at the secluded Simpsonwood conference center in Norcross, Georgia. Although the CDC convened the meeting, no public announcement was made of the gathering. Just 52 private invitations were issued. Participants included high-level officials from the CDC, FDA, top vaccine specialists from the World Health Organization, and representatives from every major vaccine manufacturer. All of the participants were repeatedly warned that the scientific data under discussion was "embargoed." Note-taking and photocopies of documents were strictly prohibited. No papers could leave the room.[41,42]

The federal health officials and industry representatives had assembled to discuss an alarming new study that confirmed a link between thimerosal (mercury) in childhood vaccines and neurological damage, including recent dramatic increases in autistic spectrum disorders. Tom Verstraeten, a CDC epidemiologist, had analyzed the agency's massive Vaccine Safety Datalink (VSD) database containing millions of medical records of vaccinated children and was "stunned" by what he saw:

> *"We have found statistically significant relationships between exposure [to mercury in vaccines] and outcomes. At two months of age, developmental delay; exposure at three months, tics; at six months, attention deficit disorder. Exposure at one, three and six months, language and speech delays—the entire category of neurodevelopmental delays."*[43,44]
> **—Dr. Tom Veerstraeten, CDC epidemiologist**

Verstraeten also discussed previous studies showing a link between mercury and neurodevelopmental disorders.[45] Since 1991, when the CDC and FDA started requiring newborn infants to receive multiple doses of thimerosal-laden hepatitis B vaccines, thimerosal-laden Hib vaccines, and the already mandated thimerosal-laden DPT and DTaP vaccines, cases of autism skyrocketed.

Dr. Bill Weil, with the American Academy of Pediatrics (AAP), told the group, "You can play with this all you want," but the results "are statistically significant."[46] Dr. Richard Johnston, an immunologist and pediatrician, exclaimed, "I do not want my grandson to get a thimerosal-containing vaccine until we know better what is going on."[47] Yet, instead of taking quick action to warn parents and recall the unsafe shots, this audacious group of 52 vaccine proponents spent the next two days calculating how to conceal the truth.[48]

"We are in a bad position from the standpoint of defending any lawsuits," said Dr. Robert Brent, a pediatrician.[49] However, Dr. Robert Chen, head of vaccine safety for the CDC, congratulated the group for their apparent success thus far at concealing the facts, and expressed relief that "given the sensitivity of the information, we have been able to keep it out of the hands of, let's say, less responsible hands."[50] Dr. John Clements, WHO vaccine advisor, was more blunt, declaring that perhaps the CDC study "should not have been done at all because the outcome could have, to some extent, been predicted." He stated that "the research results have to be handled," and warned that the study "will be taken by others and used in ways beyond the control of this group."[51]

How to "handle" undesirable scientific data:

At the Simpsonwood gathering, a new plan was devised. To begin, the CDC relinquished control of its vast database on childhood vaccines—the very same database Tom Verstraeten used to confirm a link between thimerosal-laced vaccines and autism. Although the VSD database was public property—developed at taxpayer expense—it was turned over to a private health insurance agency, ensuring that it could not be accessed by non-collaborators for additional research.[52] Three years later, Verstraeten had reworked the data and published a new version of his original study in the November 2003 issue of *Pediatrics*. However, this time "no consistent significant associations were found between thimerosal-containing vaccines and neurodevelopmental outcomes."[53]

After Simpsonwood, the CDC appeared to instruct the Institute of Medicine (IOM) to produce a new study showing no link between thimerosal and brain disorders. According to Dr. Marie McCormick, who chaired the IOM's Immunization Safety Review Committee in January 2001...

> The CDC "wants us to declare, well, that these things are pretty safe on a population basis.... We are not ever going to come down that [autism] is a true side effect" [of thimerosal].[54]
> —**Dr. Marie McCormick, Institute of Medicine**

In transcripts of the meeting, the IOM's study director, Kathleen Stratton, predicted that the IOM would conclude that the evidence was "inadequate to accept or reject a causal relation" between thimerosal and autism. Apparently, that was what "Walt wants"—a reference to Dr. Walter Orenstein, director of the CDC's National Immunization Program.[55]

The CDC sought additional "proof" that thimerosal-laced vaccines are safe. In May 2001, Dr. Gordon Douglas, then-director of strategic planning for vaccine research at the National Institutes of Health, assured a Princeton University gathering that...

> "Four current studies are taking place to rule out the proposed link between autism and thimerosal.... In order to undo the harmful effects of research claiming to link the [measles] vaccine to an elevated risk of autism, we need to conduct and publicize additional studies to assure parents of safety."[56]
> —**Gordon Douglas, MD, former president of Merck Vaccines**

Gordon Douglas formerly served as president of Merck, a major vaccine manufacturer.

Children versus profits:
On October 25, 2000, Congressman Dan Burton wrote a letter to the U.S. Health and Human Services Secretary, Donna Shalala, requesting an immediate recall of all vaccines containing thimerosal, but the FDA refused to recall any of the numerous thimerosal-containing vaccines. Instead, they suggested a phase-out over several years, permitting drug companies to continue selling their dangerous mercury-laden products to innocent children and unsuspecting parents. Doctors were encouraged to participate in this debacle.[57,58]

How safe are children in developing countries?
In May 2001, WHO committed to "develop a strong advocacy campaign to *support* the ongoing use of thimerosal."[59] In fact, the U.S. government continues to ship mercury-laden vaccines to developing countries—some of which are now experiencing dramatic increases in rates of autism. In China, where the disease was virtually unknown prior to 1999 when U.S. manufacturers introduced mercury-laced vaccines, by June 2005 there were more than 1.8 million Chinese autistics. Autistic disorders are also rising quickly in India, Nicaragua and other developing countries that are now using thimerosal-laced vaccines.[60]

Studies with conflicts of interest:
On November 30, 2002, a new study published in *The Lancet* concluded that mercury in vaccines is not harmful. However, the lead author of this study, Dr. Michael Pichichero, had a clear conflict of interest. He was paid to do other studies for Eli Lilly, the pharmaceutical company that was being sued for producing thimerosal used in vaccines.[61,62]
In October 2003, Danish researchers published a large study in the *Journal of the American Medical Association.* The authors of the study concluded that "the results do not support a causal relationship between childhood vaccination with thimerosal-containing vaccines and development of autistic spectrum disorders."[63] However, the researchers were affiliated with Statens Serum Institut, a Danish business enterprise that receives more than 80 percent of its profits from vaccines. In fact, Statens Serum Institut manufactured the thimerosal-containing pertussis vaccine that was investigated in their own study and found to be safe.[64]
On September 27, 2007, the *New England Journal of Medicine* published a study funded by the CDC. It concluded that early exposure to mercury from thimerosal-containing vaccines does not cause deficits in neuro-psychological functioning at 7 to 10 years of age. In fact, the authors of

this study claimed that babies with higher levels of mercury actually performed *better* on several tests.[65] If this study is to be believed, mercury is a well-documented neurotoxin except when it accumulates in babies by way of vaccines. Higher concentrations of mercury from vaccines apparently *improve* motor skills and cognitive dexterity.

The lead author of the study, Dr. William Thompson, was a former employee of Merck, a major manufacturer of thimerosal-containing vaccines. Other authors of the study received consulting fees, lecture fees, and/or grant support from Merck, Sanofi Pasteur, GlaxoSmithKline, MedImmune, Wyeth, Abbott, and Novartis—vaccine manufacturers with vested interests in disproving correlations between their products and debilities.[66]

Despite this study's many limitations, several statistical correlations were found between early exposure to mercury in vaccines and neuro-psychological deficits at a later age:

- Higher prenatal exposure to mercury was associated with significantly poorer performance on backward recall IQ development.
- Higher mercury exposure from birth to 7 months was associated with significantly poorer performance on behavioral regulation, and a higher likelihood of motor and speech tics.
- Higher mercury exposure during the first 28 days of life was associated with significantly poorer speech articulation.
- Among girls, increased neonatal mercury exposure was associated with significantly lower verbal IQ scores.[67]

This study also acknowledged several earlier studies that found important links between thimerosal-laden vaccines and neuropsychological deficits:

- In a previous vaccine safety analysis published in *Pediatrics,* post-neonatal exposure to thimerosal in vaccines was associated with an increased risk of language delays.[68]
- A 2004 *Pediatrics* study found that mercury from vaccines in the first year of life correlated with an increased risk of tics, a finding similar to that found in this study.[69]
- A study of 12,000 British children found an association between mercury in vaccines and poorer prosocial behavior (actions meant to benefit others or society as a whole).[70]
- Studies of prenatal exposure to methylmercury from fish intake have shown negative associations with language and spatial abilities, attention span, and dexterity.[71,72]
- Previous studies have reported negative effects of thimerosal exposure on neuronal cells, biochemical pathways, and animal behavior.[73]

The Geier thimerosal studies:

Dr. Mark Geier is a medical doctor and geneticist, a former research scientist at the National Institutes of Health, and a former professor at Johns Hopkins University. From 2003 through 2008, he and his son, David, published several studies showing a link between autistic spectrum disorders and thimerosal-containing vaccines. For example, an analysis of the federal government's Vaccine Adverse Event Reporting System (VAERS) database "showed statistical increases in the incidence rate of autism, mental retardation, and speech disorders" after children received thimerosal-containing vaccines when compared with children who received thimerosal-free vaccines. In fact, "there was a 2-fold to 6-fold increased incidence of neurodevelopmental disorders" following additional doses of mercury-containing shots.[74] A follow-up study published in the *Journal of American Physicians and Surgeons,* confirmed that children vaccinated with thimerosal-containing vaccines "have higher rates of speech disorders, autism, and heart arrest" and that "the relative risk of each of these disorders correlated with increasing doses of mercury" contained in the shots.[75]

Another study by the Geiers found that children with autism excrete significantly higher concentrations of mercury from their bodies during chelation therapy—a treatment for heavy metal poisoning—than non-autistic children.[76] Two Geier studies, published in the *Journal of Toxicology and Environmental Health,* confirmed statistical correlations between the total mercury content that children received from their vaccines and the severity of autistic symptoms.[77,78] In another study, the Geiers analyzed trends in the child immunization schedule and compared the number of autism cases and speech ailments before and after thimerosal-free vaccines were introduced. The results show that...

> *"The trends in newly diagnosed neurodevelopmental disorders correspond directly to the expansion and subsequent contraction of the cumulative mercury dose to which children were exposed from thimerosal-containing vaccines through the U.S. immunization schedule."*[79]
> —**Mark Geier, MD, PhD**

In August 2008, the *Journal of the Neurological Sciences* published a new study by Drs. Heather Young and Mark Geier that analyzed the vaccination records of more than 278,000 children during a 7-year period (1990-1996). The amount of mercury that these children received from their thimerosal-containing vaccines was compared to how often they were diagnosed with medical disorders. The study protocol was approved by the CDC. The results showed that disorders without a biologically plausible link to mercury exposure—pneumonia, congenital anomalies, and failure to thrive—did not occur at greater rates in children with greater exposure to mercury from their thimerosal-containing vaccines. In contrast, there was "a significant association between mercury exposure from thimerosal-containing vaccines and neurodevelopmental disorders"—a correlation that is biologically plausible. Infants with the most mercury from their vaccines had significantly higher rates of autism, autistic spectrum disorders, tics, attention deficit disorder, and emotional disturbances—2 to 4 times higher—when compared to infants who received less mercury from their shots.[80] [This study utilized the CDC's VSD database and confirms the original findings that led to the secret Simpsonwood gathering.]

The Generation Rescue study:

On June 26, 2007, Generation Rescue, a nonprofit institution, published the results of a study that it commissioned comparing rates of autism (and other neurological disorders) in vaccinated versus completely unvaccinated children. The $200,000 survey, conducted by SurveyUSA, an independent research firm, collected data on 17,674 children. Here is a summary of the most notable findings:

* Vaccinated boys (ages 11-17) were *112 percent* more likely to have autism, *158 percent* more likely to have a neurological disorder, and *317 percent* more likely to suffer from attention deficit hyperactivity disorder (ADHD), than unvaccinated boys.
* Vaccinated children (ages 4-17) were *120 percent* more likely to have asthma.[81,82]

Where are the autistic children at Homefirst® Health Services?

In 1973, I founded Homefirst Health Services, an alternative medical facility where babies are often delivered at home and are rarely vaccinated.

"We have a fairly large practice. We have about 30,000 or 35,000 children that we've taken care of over the years, and I don't think we have a single case of autism in children delivered by us who never received vaccines."[83]
—Mayer Eisenstein, MD, Director, Homefirst Health Services

Our patients also have significantly less asthma and diabetes compared to national rates. In the alternative medicine network which Homefirst is part of, there are virtually no cases of childhood asthma, in contrast to the overall Blue Cross rate of childhood asthma which is about 10 percent.

Where are the autistic Amish?

Dan Olmsted, a reporter for United Press International, began searching the Amish community for cases of autism. He began his quest in Lancaster County, the heart of Pennsylvania Dutch country, where statistically there should have been at least 130 people with autism.[84] However, the Amish, who still ride horse-and-buggies, also shun modern medicine and do not vaccinate their children. This may have been the reason Olmsted had a difficult time finding autistic Amish. When he finally located an Amish family with an autistic child, the mother gave the following explanation: "Unfortunately our autistic daughter, who's doing very well—she's been diagnosed with very, very severe autism—is adopted from China, and so she would have had all her vaccines in China before we got her, and then she had most of her vaccines given to her in the United States before we got her. So, we're probably not the pure case you're looking for."[85] (Photographs of the child taken in China before she was vaccinated show a smiling, alert child looking directly into the camera.)[86]

Olmsted eventually located another autistic child in the Amish community, and she was vaccinated prior to her disability as well. According to Stacey-Jean, a member of the Amish community...

> *"Almost every Amish family I know has had somebody from the health department knock on our door and try to convince us to get vaccines for our children. The younger Amish more and more are getting vaccines. It's a minority of children who vaccinate, but that is changing now. There's one family that we know; their daughter had a vaccine reaction [around 15 months of age] and is now autistic. She was walking and functioning and a happy, bright child, and 24 hours after she had her vaccine, her legs went limp and she had a typical high-pitched scream. They called the doctor and he said it was fine, that a lot of high-pitched screaming goes along with it. She completely quit speaking, quit making eye contact with people. She went into her own world."*[87]
> —**Stacey-Jean, Amish community member**

The 'better diagnosis' theory of autism:

Health authorities would like to convince parents that the rise in autism is caused by better diagnostic procedures—not vaccines. However, Dr. Boyd Haley, one of the world's foremost authorities on mercury toxicity, and head of the chemistry department at the University of Kentucky, dismisses this ruse with a logical question: "If the epidemic is truly an artifact of poor diagnosis, then where are all of the 20-year-old autistics?"[88] Dr. Haley had more to say on this topic:

You couldn't even construct a study that shows thimerosal is safe. It's just too darn toxic. If you inject thimerosal into an animal, its brain will sicken. If you apply it to living tissue, the cells die. If you put it in a petri dish, the culture dies. Knowing these things, it would be shocking if one could inject it into an infant without causing damage.[89]

—**Dr. Boyd Haley, mercury toxicity expert**

Ethylmercury (in vaccines) versus methylmercury:
Health officials often claim that ethylmercury—the type of mercury found in vaccines containing thimerosal—should not be compared to methylmercury, a well-established neurotoxin. However, a Russian study found that adults exposed to much lower concentrations of ethylmercury than those given to American children still suffered brain damage years later.[90] In 1985, the *Archives of Toxicology* published a comparative study that administered similar doses of ethylmercury and methylmercury to rats. The ethylmercury-treated rats had higher amounts of inorganic mercury in their kidneys and brains.[91] In August 2005, a study funded by the National Institutes of Health also found that ethylmercury is more toxic to the brain than methylmercury. It crosses the blood-brain barrier quicker and converts to inorganic mercury—which is more difficult to excrete and stays in the brain longer—at much higher levels.[92]

Where does the AAP stand on thimerosal in vaccines?
The American Academy of Pediatrics' (AAP) policy on mercury exposure states, "Mercury in all its forms is toxic to the fetus and children, and efforts should be made to reduce exposure to the extent possible to pregnant women and children as well as the general population."[93] Yet, the AAP supports giving pregnant women and infants flu vaccines that contain high concentrations of mercury.[94] For example, when New York state legislators considered banning thimerosal from medical products, the AAP officially opposed such legislation because it "sends the wrong message to New York parents and pregnant women, and in fact all New Yorkers."[95]

Pregnant women, infants, and mercury-laced vaccines:
In February 2006, the CDC's Advisory Committee on Immunization Practices (ACIP) repeated its recommendation that infants up to 24 months old get annual flu shots—despite containing high quantities of mercury—and even expanded its recommendation to 59 months of age! The ACIP also recommends flu vaccines for pregnant women.[96,97] In May 2007, the ACIP repeated its improbable assertion that mercury-laced flu vaccines

for pregnant women are safe.[98] The Institute of Medicine previously recommended that mercury *not* be injected into these sensitive populations.[99] Many flu shots still contain 25mcg of mercury, an amount that is considered grossly unsafe under Environmental Protection Agency (EPA) guidelines. Concerned father, Christian McIlwain, responds:

> *"Children and fetuses are still being exposed unnecessarily to this neurotoxin. With the recently added recommendations that influenza vaccines be given to women during any stage of pregnancy, and children from age 6 months and up, the amount of early-age thimerosal through recommended vaccines has increased drastically in the last two years."*[100]
> —**Christian McIlwain, concerned parent**

Clair Bothell, chair of the National Autism Association is more direct:

> *"When it comes to discussing thimerosal, it's hard to tell where the pharmaceutical industry leaves off and where the CDC begins. The blurring of these lines is not in the best interests of public health."*[101]
> —**Clair Bothell, National Autism Association**

Did autism rates improve after mercury-vaccines were stopped?
From 1999 through 2002, several vaccines with mercury were phased out of the immunization schedule. They were replaced with low-mercury, or "thimerosal-free," vaccines. Today, authorities claim that autism rates have not declined after the mercury phaseout, and use this to support their contention that vaccines are safe. (If mercury in vaccines contributed to autism, then rates should have dropped after mercury was removed.) However, during this so-called "phaseout" period, authorities actually *added* mercury-laced flu shots to the list of vaccines urged for all babies 6 to 23 months of age.[102,103] Soon thereafter, the CDC also added *pregnant women in their first trimester* to the list of people officially recommended —and actively encouraged—to receive mercury-laced flu vaccines.[104,105]

In addition to these dubious actions during this greatly publicized "phaseout" of mercury, four doses of a new vaccine with high *aluminum* content were added to the vaccine schedule (for pneumococcus).[106] Two doses of another vaccine with aluminum (for hepatitis A)[107] were added in 2005—a 20% increase in aluminum content since the mercury phaseout.[108] Thus, millions of infants in utero and babies continued to receive unnaturally high doses of neurotoxic chemicals—mercury and aluminum—long after unsuspecting parents were led to believe that vaccines were purified and made safe. (Read the chapter on aluminum for more information.)

Vaccines and Autism: Case Reports by Parents

▸ *"My beautiful, four-year-old grandson is not talking, and showing signs of autism. He was a vibrant, healthy baby, and was growing well until his baby shots at 14 months. Within a two-week period after receiving his shots, he stopped giving eye contact, turned inward, and has never been the same. He is developing well physically, but mentally and emotionally he is very delayed. My daughter suffers daily from his emotional and mental disability. It breaks my heart to see this. I don't know if he will ever be able to live a normal life. Someone committed a horrible crime against these children."*

▸ *"One day after receiving her shots, my four-year-old niece went into seizures. She slept for two days. After waking up, she had infantile behavior and was mentally challenged. She was sent to a children's hospital for physical, speech, music, and other therapies. There have been slight changes: she now mimics some words, not as much biting, but now licking things. My sister's 4-year-old is on a 1-year-old verbal level, but a 1-month-old level as far as focusing and recognizing. An infectious disease specialist said that it was probably a combination of an infection and the immunizations, but now we are being told that it was just a coincidence that she had the shots the previous day."*[109]

Vitamin D and autism:

Studies show that vitamin D might prevent some forms of cancer, protect against flu, and fight depression.[110-113] It also appears to benefit autistic children deficient in vitamin D. For example, John is a 7-year-old boy with autism. His symptoms include temper tantrums, mood swings, impaired language, digestive issues, toileting problems, and poor muscle strength. His mother noticed that his symptoms improved in the summer and regressed in the winter—a likely indication of vitamin D deficiency. (My staff performs vitamin D blood tests on our patients to determine precise vitamin D serum levels.) I advised the mother to begin John on 5,000 i.u. of vitamin D_3 per day for two weeks, followed by 2,000 i.u. per day in the form of powdered vitamin D dissolved in juice. Within one week, John's language began to return. At the end of two weeks, his language showed further improvement and he began to toilet himself. After four weeks of vitamin D treatment, the mother noted improvements in muscle strength as well as continued improvements in language.

I have treated other autistic children favorably using a similar regimen of vitamin D, often adding probiotics for digestive problems. One mother describes her experience:

"My autistic son is 12 years old. The first effect was his morning mood. He would be very agitated. I started him on 4,000 i.u. of vitamin D₃. Now he comes down to breakfast with a smile, saying 'Good morning, mama.' He is much more verbal, engaged, and doing better with his school work. He is not 'cured' but we are in a better place. His fits have decreased in number and intensity. The probiotics changed his life as well. His seasonal asthma diminished since he started to use them. Thank you."
—**Mother of an autistic child**

Another mother describes her experience:

"Dear Dr. Eisenstein, prior to seeing you, my 5-year-old autistic son was very aggressive, head-butting other children, bruising his teacher. I wondered what will happen 5 or 10 years from now when he is bigger and stronger than me, when he has a meltdown and becomes aggressive. Will I fear for my life? One month after you started him on 5,000 i.u. of vitamin D, he is focused, engaging, happy, and laughing appropriately. He is less aggressive. He is vocalizing, and seems to be picking things up easier. His understanding is better than before. Thank you so much for what you have done to make our whole family's quality of life better."[114]
—**Mother of an autistic child**

Of course, vitamin D is just a one healthcare option—an inexpensive first line of remediation. Autistic children require professional analysis, testing, support, and a multifaceted treatment strategy.

Notes

1. Kanner, Leo. "Autistic disturbances of affective content." *The Nervous Child II* (1942-1943):250.

2. Treffert, DA. "Epidemiology of infantile autism." *Archives of General Psychiatry* (May 1970);22(5):431-38.

3. Lotter, V. "Epidemiology of autistic conditions in young children, I. Prevalence." *Social Psychiatry* 1966; 1:24-37.

4. American Psychiatric Association. *Diagnostic and Statistical Manual of Mental Disorders,* Third Edition, Revised, (Washington, DC, 1987):36-37.

5. CDC. "Autism prevalence." www.hhs.gov

6. Rice, C., et al. "Prevalence of autism spectrum disorders—autism and developmental disabilities monitoring network, six sites, United States, 2000; 14 sites, United States, 2002." *MMWR CDC Surveillance Summaries* (February 9, 2007);56(SS-1).

7. Kogan, MD., et al. "Prevalence of parent-reported diagnosis of autism spectrum disorder (ASD) among children in the U.S., 2007." *Pediatrics* (October 5, 2009).

8. Tsouderos, T. "Proportion of 8-year-olds diagnosed with autism is up 50% in 2 years, CDC says." *LA Times* (October 5, 2009).

9. U.S. Autism and Asperger Association, Inc. "S. 843 Combating Autism Act passed by United States House of Representatives; landmark legislation to help scientists understand the causes and characteristics of autism." *Special Edition* (December 6, 2006).

10. Ibid.

11. Kanner, Leo. "To what extent is early infantile autism determined by constitutional inadequacies?" *Genetics & the Inheritance of Integrated Neurological and Psychiatric Patterns,* (Baltimore: Williams and Wilkins, 1954):382.

12. Kanner, Leo, et al., "Early infantile autism: 1943-1955," *Psych Res Reports* 1957;7:62.

13. Kanner, Leo. "Early infantile autism," *J of Pediatrics* 1944;25:217.

14. Gillberg, C., et al. "Social class and infantile autism," *J of Autism* 1982; 12(3):223.

15. Coulter, Harris. *Vaccination, Social Violence, and Criminality: Medical Assault on the American Brain,* (Berkeley, CA: North Atlantic, 1990).

16. "Autism: Present Challenges, Future Needs—Why the Increased Rates?" *Government Reform Committee Hearing,* Washington, DC. (April 6, 2000.)

17. Ibid. As coted in the testimony of Coleen Boyle, PhD.

18. Fudenberg, HH. "Dialysable lymphocyte extract (DlyE) in infantile onset autism: pilot study." *Biotherapy* 1996;9:143-7.

19. Gupta, S. "Immunology and immunologic treatment of autism." *Proc of Natl Autism Assoc, Chicago* 1996;455-60.

20. Statement by Bernard Rimland at the National Autism Conference in Chicago sponsored by the *Autism Research Institute* (June 1996).

21. Yazbak, FE. "Autism: Is there a vaccine connection? Part I. Vaccination after delivery." 1999. www.garynull.com/documents/autism99b.htm

22. Yazbak, FE. "Autism: Is there a vaccine connection? Part II. Vaccination around pregnancy." 1999. www.garynull.com/documents/autism99b2.htm

23. Yazbak, FE. "Autism: Is there a vaccine connection? Part III. Vaccination around pregnancy, the sequel." 2000. www.garynull.com/documents/autism99b3.htm

24. Institute of Medicine. "Immunization safety review: measles-mumps-rubella vaccine and autism." (Washington, DC: National Academy Press, 2001).

25. In a copy of Dan Burton's letter to President Bush.

26. Zwillich, T. "U.S. government asks court to seal vaccine records." *Reuters Health* (November 26, 2002).

27. Gillers, S. "Why judges should make court documents public." *NY Times* (November 30, 2002).

28. Corrigan, S. "MMR fears coming true." *Mail on Sunday* (February 5, 2006). www.dailymail.co.uk

29. Palta, R. "A timeline of the thimerosal controversy." *Mother Jones* (March 1, 2004).

30. FDA. "Thimerosal as a preservative." www.fda.gov

31. Legal Rights. "Thimerosal & autism symptoms resource: dangers of mercury." www.thimerosal-autism-symptoms.com/html/mercury.html (Aug 11, 2009.)

32. Wikipedia. "Thimerosal." www.en.wikipedia.org/wiki/thimerosal

33. Levin, M. "'91 memo warned of mercury in vaccines." *L.A. Times* (Feb 8, 2005):A-1.

34. AAP/PHS. "Joint statement of the American Academy of Pediatrics (AAP) and the United States Public Health Service (PHS)," (July 7, 1999).

35. A-Champ. "CDC failure to remove mercury from vaccines." *Advocates for Children's Health Affected by Mercury Poisoning.*" www.a-champ.org/cdcmercuryremoval.html (May 10, 2007).

36. Kennedy, RF. "Time for CDC to come clean." *Huffington Post* (March 1, 2006).

37. Ibid.

38. Ibid.

39. Ibid.

40. Olmsted, D. "Autism and the Homefirst® medical practice. The age of autism: a pretty big secret." *United Press International* (Dec. 7, 2005). www.homefirst.com

41. Data accessed via the Freedom of Information Act.

42. Kennedy, RF. "Deadly immunity." *Common Dreams NewsCenter* (June 21, 2005). Originally published by *Salon.com* (June 16, 2005). Updates to the story were made on June 17, June 22, June 24, July 1 and July 21, 2007.

43. National Autism Association. From transcripts of the meeting (via FOIA). Received in an email dated June 28, 2006.

44. See Notes 41 and 42.

45. See Notes 41-43.

46. Ibid.

47. Ibid.
48. Ibid.
49. Ibid.
50. Ibid.
51. Ibid.
52. See Note 42.
53. Verstraeten, T., et al. "Safety of thimerosal-containing vaccines: a two-phased study of computerized health maintenance organization databases." *Pediatrics* (Nov 2003); 112(5):1039-48.
54. See Note 42.
55. Ibid.
56. Ibid.
57. As noted in a copy of the original letter. www.altcorp.com/repburton.htm
58. Press release. "Chairman Burton requests vaccine recall," (Oct. 26, 2000).
59. See Note 36.
60. See Note 42.
61. Pichichero, M., et al. "Mercury concentrations and metabolism in infants receiving vaccines containing thimerosal." *The Lancet* (November 30, 2002);360(9347):1737-41.
62. McNeil, D. "Study suggests mercury in vaccine was not harmful." *NY Times* (December 4, 2002).
63. Hviid, A., et al. "Association between thimerosal-containing vaccine and autism." *JAMA* 2003;290:1763-1766.
64. Rimland, B. "To the editor, re: Association between thimerosal-containing vaccine and autism." *J of the American Medical Association* (January 14, 2004).
65. Thompson, W., et al. "Early thimerosal exposure and neuropsychological outcomes at 7 to 10 years." *NEJM* (September 27, 2007); 357:1281-92.
66. Ibid.
67. Ibid.
68. See Note 53.
69. Andrews, N., et al. "Thimerosal exposure in infants and developmental disorders: a retrospective cohort study in the United Kingdom does not support a causal association." *Pediatrics* 2004;114:584-91.
70. Heron, J., et al. "Thimerosal exposure in infants and developmental disorders: a prospective cohort study in the United Kingdom does not support a causal association." *Pediatrics* 2004:114:577-83.
71. Grandjean, P., et al. "Methymercury exposure biomarkers as indicators of neurotoxicity in children aged 7 years." *Amer J Epidemiology* 1999;150:301-305.
72. Crump, KS., et al. "Influence of prenatal mercury exposure upon scholastic and psychological test performance: benchmark analysis of a New Zealand cohort." *Risk Anal* 1998;18 701-13.
73. See Note 65, references 22-31.
74. Geier, M. and Geier, D. "Neurodevelopmental disorders after thimerosal-containing vaccines: a brief communication." *Exper Bio Med* 2003;228:660-64.
75. Geier, M. and Geier, D. "Thimerosal in childhood vaccines, neuro-developmental disorders, and heart disease in the United States." *Journal of American Physicians and Surgeons* 2003;8(1):6-11.
76. Bradstreet, J., Geier, D., et al. "A case-control study of mercury burden in children with autistic spectrum disorders." *J of American Physicians and Surgeons* 2003;8(3):76-79.
77. Geier, M. and Geier, D. "A case series of children with apparent mercury toxic encephalopathies manifesting with clinical symptoms of regressive autistic disorders." *Journal of Toxicology and Environmental Health,* Part A: Current Issues (April 30, 2007).
78. Geier, M. and Geier, D. "A prospective study of mercury toxicity biomarkers in autistic spectrum disorders." *J of Tox and Envir Health,* 2007; Part A, Vol 70(20):1723-30.
79. Geier, M. and Geier, D. "Early downward trends in neurodevelopmental disorders following removal of thimerosal-containing vaccines." *Journal of American Physicians and Surgeons* 2006;11(1):8-13.
80. Young, HA, Geier, M., et al. "Thimerosal exposure in infants and neuro-developmental disorders: an assessment of computerized medical records in the Vaccine Safety Datalink." *J Neurol Sci* (August 15, 2008);271(1-2):110-18.

81. Handley, JB. "Cal-Oregon unvaccinated survey." *Generation Rescue* (June 26, 2007). www.generationrescue.org/survey.html

82. Olmsted, D. "The age of autism: study sees vaccine risk." *Sci Daily* (June 26, 2007).

83. Eisenstein, M. Homefirst Health Services. www.homefirst.com

84. Olmsted, D. "The age of autism: the Amish anomaly." *United Press International* (April 18, 2005).

85. Olmsted, D. "The age of autism: Julia." *United Press International* (April 19, 2005).

86. Ibid.

87. Ibid.

88. See Note 42.

89. Ibid.

90. Ibid.

91. Magos, L., et al. "The comparative toxicology of ethyl- and methylmercury." *Archives of Toxicology* 1985;57:260-67.

92. Burbacher, TM., et al. "Comparison of blood and brain levels in infant monkeys exposed to methylmercury or vaccines containing thimerosal." *Environ Health Perspect* 2005;113(8): 1015-21.

93. National Autism Association. "American Academy of Pediatrics (AAP) devotes little time to autism epidemic at October convention." Press release: September 19, 2005.

94. Department of Health and Human Services/CDC. "Recommended immunization schedule for ages 0-6 years, United States, 2010." The immunization schedule is approved by the CDC (ACIP) and the American Academy of Pediatrics (AAP).

95. See Note 93.

96. CDC. *Morbidity and Mortality Weekly Report,* 2007;56(9):193-196.

97. CDC. *Morbidity and Mortality Weekly Report,* (July 28, 2006);55(10).

98. CDC. "Guidelines for vaccinating pregnant women." www.cdc.gov (May 2007).

99. FDA. "Table 3: Thimerosal and expanded list of vaccines." www.fda.gov (Updated: March 14, 2008.)

100. National Autism Association. "Controversial vaccine preservative to be discussed at upcoming CDC meeting: parents and advocacy groups request flu shots recommended for pregnant women, infants and children be mercury-free." Press release: Feb 14, 2007.

101. National Autism Association. "CDC's vaccine committee whitewashed toxic vaccine component, says National Autism Association." Press release: February 23, 2007.

102. AAP News. "Flu vaccine extended to kids 6-23 months." *American Academy of Pediatrics* (August 2002).

103. "Childhood influenza-vaccination coverage—United States, 2002-03 influenza season." *JAMA* 2004;292: 2074-75.

104. Bettes, B., et al. "Influenza vaccination in pregnancy: practices among obstetrician-gynecologists—US, 2003-04 influenza season" (editorial note). *Medscape* (Oct 28, 2005).

105. CDC. "Prevention and control of influenza: recommendations of the ACIP." *MMWR* 2005;54(41):1050-52.

106. CDC. "Preventing pneumococcal disease among infants and young children." *MMWR* 2000;49(RR09):1-38.

107. CDC. "CDC's ACIP expands hepatitis A vaccination for children." *Press Release* (October 28, 2005).

108. [Prior to the mercury phaseout (pre-2000), babies received 3,925mcg of aluminum by 18 months of age. After Prevnar and hepatitis A shots were added to the schedule, babies received 4,925mcg of aluminum by 18 months of age—a 20% increase.]

109. Thinktwice Global Vaccine Institute. Unsolicited case reports submitted by concerned parents. www.thinktwice.com

110. Goodwin, PJ. "Vitamin D in cancer patients." *J Clin Oncology* (May 1, 2009):2117-19.

111. Cannell JJ, et al. "Epidemic influenza and vitamin D." *Epidemiology and Infection* 2006;134:1129–40.

112. Murphy, PK., et al. "Vitamin D and mood disorders among women." *J of Midwifery and Women's Health* (Sep-Oct 2008);53(5):440-446.

113. Cannell, JJ. "Vitamin D and your health: autism." *Vitamin D Council* (February 2, 2009). www.vitamindcouncil.org

114. Homefirst Health Services. Case reports submitted by patients of Dr. Eisenstein. www.homefirst.com

Chickenpox

What is chickenpox?

Chickenpox, or varicella, is a contagious disease caused by a virus. The technical name for this virus is varicella-zoster, a member of the herpes virus family. Chickenpox is considered by many experts to be a relatively harmless childhood ailment:

"Chickenpox is generally a benign, self-limiting disease."[1]
—Merck, chickenpox vaccine manufacturer

Symptoms include a fever, runny nose, sore throat, and an itchy skin rash which can appear anywhere on the body. The rash and disease usually disappear after one or two weeks. The disease usually confers permanent immunity; it is rarely contracted again.

Is chickenpox dangerous?

Chickenpox can be itchy and uncomfortable for a few days. Serious problems are rare. In fact, before a chickenpox vaccine was introduced, doctors recommended exposing children to the virus, and parents organized "chickenpox parties" because complication rates increase when the disease is contracted by teenagers or adults.[2] Prior to the introduction of the chickenpox vaccine, of the millions of people in the United States who contracted this disease every year, about 100 died from related complications.[3] Many of these fatalities were in adults who did not have chickenpox as a child, or in previously unhealthy children—youngsters with already weakened immune systems from other diseases, such as AIDS, leukemia, or cancer.[4]

History of the chickenpox vaccine:

A chickenpox vaccine has been available since the 1970s but authorities were reluctant to license and promote it because the disease is rarely dangerous and confers lifelong immunity. However, the vaccine contains a weakened form of the virus; once injected, it remains in the body indefinitely.[5] Authorities were concerned that it could reawaken years after the vaccination and cause serious problems. Also, if immunity from the vaccine were to prove temporary, like other vaccines, children who are prevented from contracting the disease naturally, due to widespread use of the shot, might become more susceptible to chickenpox during adulthood when the disease can be serious.

Quick Facts About Chickenpox

♦ **Chickenpox is usually a harmless, childhood ailment.** Serious problems are rare.

♦ **Chickenpox usually confers permanent immunity.** It is rarely contracted again.

♦ **Complications from chickenpox mainly occur in adults who did not have chickenpox as a child, or in previously unhealthy children** —like those with already weakened immune systems from other diseases, such as AIDS, leukemia, or cancer.

The chickenpox vaccine was originally developed for children with leukemia or weak immune systems, a small population at greater risk for complications from the disease.[6] But the vaccine manufacturer sought a wider market for its lucrative product. Merck invested millions of dollars in this vaccine, and according to Samuel Katz, Chairman of Pediatrics at Duke University, and head of a vaccine committee at the National Academy of Sciences...

"Merck isn't going to make back its investment in that vaccine by just distributing it to kids with cancer. They're going to be interested in pushing for use in the normal population."[7]
—Samuel Katz, MD, Chairman of Pediatrics, Duke University

A study conducted in 1985 by the Centers for Disease Control and Prevention (CDC) determined that the medical costs of treating chickenpox did not warrant spending the money on a national vaccination campaign.[8] However, a few years later authorities came up with a new rationale to license this vaccine. It was now being touted as "cost-effective" when the indirect expenses of missed work and school time are factored in.[9,10] In other words, the chickenpox vaccine was not being promoted as essential, but rather as money-saving, because moms and dads would no longer have to stay home (an average of one day) to care for their sick children.[11]

The chickenpox vaccine:
- Varivax—A live-virus vaccine designed to protect against varicella. The virus "was initially obtained from a child with natural varicella, then introduced into human embryonic lung cell cultures, adapted to and propagated in embryonic guinea pig cell cultures, and finally

propagated in human diploid cell cultures" (fetal tissue). Each dose contains "a minimum of 1350 PFU (plaque forming units) of Oka/Merck varicella virus," plus sodium chloride, sodium phosphate, potassium phosphate, potassium chloride, hydrolyzed gelatin, monosodium L-glutamate (MSG), sucrose, and "residual components of MRC-5 cells including DNA and protein...EDTA, neomycin (an antibiotic), and fetal bovine serum." Produced by Merck. U.S. licensed in 1995. Given in 2 doses.[12]

Safety

The CDC and FDA recently analyzed more than 6,500 adverse reactions to the chickenpox vaccine that occurred during a period of less than 3½ years. Their findings were published in the *Journal of the American Medical Association*.[13] Here is a summary of their findings:

- Adverse reactions in recipients of the chickenpox vaccine occurred at a rate of 67.5 per 100,000 doses sold.
- Approximately 4 percent of reports described "serious" adverse reactions. (By FDA definition, *serious* reactions refer to deaths, life-threatening events, hospitalizations, persistent or significant disabilities, and other incidents of medical importance. For example, the data analyzed in this study included numerous cases of neurological disorders, immune system damage, blood disorders, brain inflammation, seizures, and death.)
- Children under 4 years of age had *serious* reactions at a rate of 6.3 percent.
- Children under 2 years of age had *serious* reactions at a rate of 9.2 percent.
- Children vaccinated (by mistake) between birth and their first birthday had *serious* reactions at an astonishing rate of 14 percent!
- These figures do not take into account that "doses sold" is a CDC "projection" for which no reliable documentation can be found. Authors of the study based their figures on oral and private "unpublished data" from the CDC. In some parts of the country vaccination rates were below 10 percent. Therefore, the true rate of adverse reactions associated with the chickenpox vaccine could be much higher.
- The FDA admitted that "potentially substantial underreporting" made the figures "highly variable fractions of actual event numbers."

The FDA and CDC findings included a few case histories.[14] For example:

▸ One healthy 18-month-old boy who "had no history of allergy or any prior post-vaccinal adverse event" before he received the chickenpox vaccine (along with others), was admitted to the intensive care unit four days later with a low platelet count. "He began to bleed from the mouth...and died two days later from cerebral hemorrhage."

▸ Another child "without previous convulsions" had an absence seizure three days after varicella vaccine. Following his second dose one month later, he reacted with two generalized tonic-clonic seizures. The researchers noted, "This patient's positive rechallenge for seizure activity *increases suspicion that varicella vaccine may be more than a coincidental factor in observations of postvaccinal convulsions*" [author's emphasis added].

▸ A four-year-old girl developed hemiparesis (partial paralysis on one side of the body) two weeks after receiving the chickenpox vaccine. Medical investigators concluded that "her apparent cerebrovascular accident assumes particular importance after a recent description of a significant statistical association between natural chickenpox and subsequent ischemic strokes in children." [Interpretation: researchers believe that the vaccine caused her serious disorder.]

Can the chickenpox vaccine cause SHINGLES?

The FDA and CDC findings also include numerous reports of vaccine recipients developing herpes zoster, or shingles, a painful skin eruption that can last for several weeks. This affliction can occur again and again, months or years following the shot. Once the varicella virus is injected into the body, it remains there indefinitely and can reactivate when immunity declines. According to Dr. Dennis Klinman of the FDA Center for Biologics Evaluation and Research, and author of a pertinent study published in *Nature Medicine,* reactivation of the dormant infection can occur following inoculation with the live virus chickenpox vaccine: "As immunity declines, the latent virus wakes up."[15,16] Earlier studies published in both the *New England Journal of Medicine* and the *Pediatric Infectious Disease Journal* also showed this link between the chickenpox vaccine and herpes zoster.[17,18]

The following case reports were provided by doctors.[19,20] They are typical of the many children who are afflicted with shingles after temporary immunity from their chickenpox vaccine declines with time.

▸ A 15-month old baby received the chickenpox vaccine and 3 months later developed painful, blistering lesions on his right shoulder, arm and hand. He also had a patch of blisters on the right-center of his back. The child was diagnosed with shingles by his doctor.

‣ A 2-year-old boy received the chickenpox vaccine. At the age of 5 years, he had a painful shingles eruption on the back of his neck that lasted for 45 days. Nine months later, he had another outbreak of shingles on his left nipple and the left side of his back. The pain was severe and the rash left scars. Two months later, he had yet another shingles outbreak.

‣ A 4-year-old girl received the chickenpox vaccine and 5 months later developed painful "grouped vesicles" that extended down the back of her arm. The child was diagnosed with shingles by her pediatrician.

Shingles in the non-vaccinated population:

As shown above, the chickenpox vaccine can cause shingles in some children who receive the vaccine. However, it is also indirectly responsible for shingles outbreaks in older people who never received the vaccine —adults who contracted chickenpox naturally as children. These people rely on natural varicella circulating throughout society. They gain an antibody boost that protects them against shingles whenever they periodically come into contact with natural, airborne chickenpox. Today, with fewer cases of wild chickenpox circulating in the community, this is less and less likely. According to Dr. James Cherry, a professor of pediatrics at Mattel Children's Hospital at the University of California, Los Angeles...

"Our immunity is stimulated by being exposed to the chickenpox. When that stimulation goes away, our protection is going to decrease, so we'll see more cases of shingles. My guess is that we're going to be giving doses of the [chickenpox] vaccine to 30- and 40-year-olds to prevent shingles. The better we do in [eradicating chickenpox], the more we're going to see shingles."[21]
—James Cherry, MD, professor of pediatrics

Dr. Gary Goldman, an expert varicella research analyst hired by the CDC in 1995 to collect data and monitor trends associated with the newly introduced chickenpox vaccine, is even more candid:

"The universal varicella vaccination program in the United States...will leave our population vulnerable to shingles epidemics. There appears to be no way to avoid a mass epidemic of shingles lasting as long as several generations among adults."[22,23]
—Gary Goldman, PhD, expert varicella research analyst

The CDC, FDA, and vaccine manufacturer may have traded a relatively mild childhood disease—chickenpox—for a much more serious ailment.[24] In fact, *shingles causes five times as many hospitalizations and three times as many deaths as chickenpox.*[25] (The FDA recently licensed a new shingles vaccine, Zostavax, manufactured by Merck, the same company that developed Varivax, the chickenpox vaccine that may be indirectly *causing* epidemics of shingles. In other words, a new vaccine was produced to treat a problem exacerbated by an earlier vaccine.)

Can vaccinated children spread chickenpox to other people?

Product inserts from the chickenpox vaccine manufacturer contain a warning that vaccinated individuals—"healthy vaccinees"—may transmit the vaccine virus to family and friends—"healthy susceptible contacts"—and that vaccine recipients "should attempt to avoid, whenever possible, close association with susceptible high-risk individuals for up to six weeks," such as newborns, pregnant women, and people with compromised immune systems.[26] The *Journal of Pediatrics* published a study confirming that children vaccinated against chickenpox can spread the disease, often with disastrous consequences. For example, a pregnant woman who caught chickenpox from her vaccinated son chose to abort the fetus rather than risk giving birth to a prenatally-injured baby.[27] Chickenpox vaccine data reported to the federal government (VAERS) includes many cases of these "unintentional exposures."[28] The CDC and FDA also admit that "secondary transmission of the virus can occur."[29] In other words, *children vaccinated with the chickenpox shot are mobile carriers of the virus, and can spread this highly contagious disease to every susceptible person they come into contact with.*

The chickenpox vaccine shifted the disease to older age groups:

Prior to licensing the chickenpox vaccine, the *American Journal of Epidemiology* published a theoretical study showing that mass vaccination would shift the age distribution of chickenpox cases from children, who are unlikely to have problems with this disease, to teenagers and adults, who have higher complication rates.[30] In fact, *adults are 10 times more likely to require hospitalization and 25 times more likely to die from chickenpox than children.*[31] Yet, this did not stop authorities from licensing and mandating this vaccine. In response, Dr. William Osheroff, medical director of Pacificare Health Systems, a large Health Management Organization (HMO), chose not to recommend Varivax. He correctly summarized the pertinent issues:

"This is a very benign disease in children but the vaccine may create a false sense of security as these children get older and find themselves non-immune. Chickenpox as an adult is a serious disease."[32]
—**William Osheroff, MD, medical director of a large HMO**

The *New England Journal of Medicine* recently confirmed that the vaccine shifted demographics over time. Before the vaccine was introduced, most cases of chickenpox occurred in children between 3 and 6 years of age. By 2004, just 30 percent of cases were in children under the age of 6 years. Older people are now more susceptible.[33]

Additional confirmation of adverse reactions:
Common reactions that have been reported following chickenpox vaccination include upper and lower respiratory illness, gastrointestinal disorders, ear infection, eye complaints, swollen lymph nodes, headache, muscle pain, joint pain, fatigue, malaise, disturbed sleep, loss of appetite, diarrhea, vomiting, and a chickenpox-like rash on the body (often occurring within a few days to three or four weeks following the shot).[34]

Serious reactions that have been reported following chickenpox vaccination include anaphylaxis (a sudden, severe, and potentially fatal allergic reaction), thrombocytopenia (a dangerous blood disorder), Henoch-Schönlein purpura (inflammation of the blood vessels), encephalitis (inflammation of the brain), transverse myelitis (inflammation of the spinal cord), Guillain-Barré syndrome (muscle weakness and paralysis), Bell's palsy (facial paralysis), seizures, aseptic meningitis (inflammation of the tissues that cover the brain), Stevens-Johnson syndrome (a potentially deadly skin disease), pneumonia, pharyngitis (inflammation of the pharynx), secondary bacterial infections, and herpes zoster (shingles).[35]

Although many parents are unaware that the chickenpox vaccine can cause serious adverse reactions in their children, some make the connection. For example, one mother wrote the following:

"My five-year-old son received the chickenpox vaccine. Two weeks later I took him to the doctor because I noticed a lot of bruising. Four days later I took him back to the doctor for blood work. That evening I was instructed to rush him to the children's hospital. He was diagnosed with thrombocytopenia and had to have intravenous immunoglobulin transfusions. Two months later his platelets skyrocketed then dropped. This is related to the chickenpox vaccine because he showed no other virus or illness prior to his diagnosis."[36]
—**Concerned mother of a chickenpox-vaccinated child**

Chickenpox Vaccine: VAERS Case Reports

▸107121: A 1-year-old child developed a rash, vomited, let out a shrill scream, went into cardiac arrest and died, four days after getting the chickenpox vaccine.

▸158878: A 14-month-old baby girl acquired chickenpox one day after receiving the chickenpox vaccine. Two days later she developed cellulitis that required hospitalization and surgery on her labia.

▸279453: A 15-month-old baby developed life-threatening respiratory distress after receiving the chickenpox vaccine. Hospitalization was required.

▸131631: A 2-year-old baby became dazed and passed out approximately five minutes after receiving the chickenpox vaccine.

▸87553: A 2-year-old baby developed pericarditis, vasculitis, liver damage, and swollen lips two weeks after her chickenpox shot. She was hospitalized.

▸79983: A 2-year-old baby developed acute autoimmune hemolytic anemia 12 days after receiving the chickenpox vaccine. Hospitalization was required.

▸121661: A 3-year-old child received the chickenpox vaccine. Nine days later he was paralyzed, unable to walk or urinate.

▸106164: A 4-year-old child developed a "varicella-like rash" six days after his chickenpox vaccine, and was hospitalized with staphylococcal bacteremia.

▸122210: A 4-year-old child developed kidney damage two days after receiving the chickenpox vaccine. Two weeks later, she contracted chickenpox and a superinfection. Hospitalization was required.

▸80082: A 4-year-old child developed lymphocytic leukemia, headaches, leg pain, bruises, and decreased hemoglobin and platelet counts starting the day after his chickenpox vaccine. He was hospitalized for 28 days.

▸88834: A 5-year-old child developed vasculitis and Stevens-Johnson syndrome five weeks after her chickenpox vaccine. She required 10 days in the hospital.

▸175928: An 8-year-old child became dizzy and confused three days after receiving the chickenpox vaccine. The child developed seizures and was life-flighted to the hospital.

▸275714: An 8-year-old boy vomited and lost consciousness 10 minutes after receiving the chickenpox vaccine. He was unresponsive, diagnosed with acute respiratory distress, and rushed to the emergency room.

▸218460: A 9-year-old girl developed Guillain-Barré syndrome after receiving the chickenpox vaccine. She spent five weeks in the hospital.

▸114146: A 9-year-old child developed a serious blood disorder 13 days after receiving the chickenpox vaccine. Hospitalization was required.

▸219497: Four days after receiving the chickenpox vaccine, this child became unresponsive, developed a focal seizure and started foaming at the mouth. Hospitalization was required.

▸90120: A 12-year-old child developed Guillain-Barré syndrome 12 days after receiving the chickenpox vaccine.

Numerous adverse reaction reports pertaining to Varivax continue to be filed with the federal government. Many of the serious ailments—often requiring an emergency room visit and/or prolonged hospitalization—are commonly recognized complications of natural chickenpox thoroughly documented in the medical literature. Thus, as the FDA has noted in its earlier analysis, they "bolster suspicions of relationships with" and are "plausible as potential effects of" the chickenpox vaccine.[37]

The case reports on the previous page were taken directly from the FDA's Vaccine Adverse Event Reporting System (VAERS).[38] They are just a small sample of the potential harm associated with this vaccine.

Efficacy

The chickenpox vaccine manufacturer claims that its vaccine has "an estimated efficacy of 94 percent" in children after one dose—but only when "compared with the age-adjusted expected incidence rates in susceptible subjects over the same period."[39] The manufacturer claims that its vaccine is 98 percent effective in children after two doses.[40] It should be noted that each dose of the chickenpox vaccine contains approximately 1350 units of the chickenpox virus (designed to stimulate an antibody response). However, in the clinical studies used to measure the vaccine's efficacy, a much stronger vaccine was tested on children—one containing up to 17,000 units of the chickenpox virus. In fact, the vaccine manufacturer admits that "no placebo-controlled trial was carried out with Varivax using the current vaccine."[41] This means that the vaccine is unlikely to be as effective as advertised.

Vaccine Failures: In all pre-licensure trials, some vaccinated children contracted chickenpox.[42,43] Vaccine failures and/or the development of a rash virtually identical to chickenpox, account for many of the documented (and undocumented) complaints associated with this shot.[44] According to an FDA report, about 1 in 10 vaccinated children develop "breakthrough" disease following exposure to chickenpox.[45] Actual statistics are worse because some people do not report their reactions, and because vaccinated children who contract shingles or some other disease as a result of the shot are not listed as recipients of an ineffective or failed vaccine.

Although many parents are unaware that the chickenpox vaccine can actually *cause* chickenpox (or shingles) in their children, some make the connection. For example, one mother wrote the following:

"My twins were immunized with the chickenpox vaccine. Ever since they received the shot, they have had a recurring rash that looks like chickenpox. It first showed up three days after vaccinations. Nothing works to treat the bumps. The bumps are concentrated in one area, typical of shingles. Our doctors deny it, so basically we just have to deal with this. I wish I had never vaccinated them against chickenpox. My other children caught chickenpox naturally and it never hurt any of them. Please pass this letter on to others who are considering this vaccine so they can make a better decision."[46]

—**Concerned mother of two chickenpox-vaccinated children**

In March 2007, the *New England Journal of Medicine* published a study that examined ten years of chickenpox vaccine data in 350,000 subjects to assess the "loss of vaccine-induced immunity to varicella over time."[47] A few important points were made:

- The annual rate of "breakthrough" varicella (cases of chickenpox that occur in people who were vaccinated against chickenpox) significantly increased with time since vaccination.
- Nearly 10 percent of all chickenpox cases were breakthrough disease.
- Children who had been vaccinated at least five years previously, were twice as likely to have moderate-to-severe disease (when compared with more recently vaccinated children). Severe disease refers to ailments such as pneumonia and skin superinfections.
- Waning of immunity may result in increased susceptibility later in life, when the risk of severe complications is greater than that in childhood.

Additional considerations:
- The chickenpox vaccine is not effective in babies under 12 months.
- Studies indicate that the chickenpox vaccine may be less effective in children when given in combination with other vaccines.
- The vaccine appears to have reduced the number of natural chickenpox cases in society. However, regular exposure to wild chickenpox stimulates varicella antibodies and may be essential to sustain immunity. According to the manufacturer, "the duration of protection from varicella obtained using Varivax in the absence of wild-type boosting is unknown."[48]
- The vaccine manufacturer acknowledges that "there are insufficient data to assess the rate of protection against the complications of chickenpox (e.g., encephalitis, hepatitis, pneumonia) in children."[49]

The Chickenpox Vaccine and Pregnant Women

In order to avoid the risk of birth defects, pregnant women should not receive this vaccine nor come into close contact with a recently vaccinated child. In addition, women should not become pregnant for three months after receiving this vaccine.[50]

Is the chickenpox vaccine required?

Despite numerous concerns about safety and efficacy, this vaccine has been added to the growing list of mandatory shots. Dr. John Close, a California-based medical practitioner, is wary of this vaccine:

"The list of those who would constitute high-risk individuals is fairly extensive.... I have seen reports of serious adverse reactions up to four percent.... I have not found any reliable reports assessing the completeness of immunity conferred.... Of all the vaccines available at this point, this is the one I would be reluctant to make mandatory."[51]
—**John Close, MD, family practice physician**

Concerns about the vaccine's waning efficacy over time, and the increasing number of older people who are becoming more susceptible to the disease, have impelled authorities to fiddle with chickenpox vaccine recommendations. Two doses are now advocated for most people. In addition, healthcare providers have "standing orders" to ensure that women without evidence of immunity to chickenpox who have recently given birth, or have otherwise terminated a pregnancy, are vaccinated before discharge from the facility.[52] Complete chickenpox vaccine guidelines are published by the CDC. Of course, legal exemptions are permitted. Read your state vaccine laws for more information.

Notes

1. Merck & Co., Inc. "Varivax [Varicella Virus Vaccine Live (Oka/Merck)]." Product insert from the vaccine manufacturer (Issued: June 2009).
2. National Network for Immunization Information. "Exposure parties: chickenpox parties." www.immunizationinfo.org (Last visited: August 11, 2009).
3. Preblud, SR. "Varicella: complications and costs." *Pediatrics* 1986;78:728-735.
4. Ibid.
5. Gorman, Christine. "Chickenpox Conundrum." *Time* (July 19, 1993):53.
6. National Vaccine Information Center. "The Vaccine Reaction" (May 1995). www.909shot.com
7. Wessel, D. "Long incubation: A vaccine to prevent chickenpox is near; now, will

it be used?" *Wall Street Journal* (January 16, 1985):1.

8. See Note 5.

9. Lieu, TA., et al. "Cost-effectiveness of a routine varicella vaccination program for U.S. children." *Journal of the American Medical Association* 1994;271:375-81.

10. Medical Sciences Bulletin. "Chickenpox vaccine approved" (April 1995).

11. Sullivan-Bolyai, JZ., et al. "Impact of chickenpox on households of healthy children." *Pediatric Infectious Disease Journal* 1987;6:33-35.

12. See Note 1.

13. Wise, RP., et al. "Postlicensure safety surveillance for varicella vaccine." *Journal of the American Medical Association* (September 13, 2000):1271-79.

14. Ibid.

15. Klinman, D., et al. "Varicella vaccination: evidence for frequent reactivation of the vaccine strain in healthy children." *Nature Medicine* 2000;6:451-54.

16. McKinney, M. "Varicella zoster vaccine reactivates when immunity declines." *Reuters Health* (March 29, 2000).

17. Plotkin, S. "Hell's fire and varicella-vaccine safety." *New England Journal of Medicine* 1988;318:573-75.

18. Kohl, S., et al. "Natural varicella-zoster virus reactivation shortly after varicella immunization in a child." *Pediatric Infectious Disease J* 1999; 18:1112-13.

19. Goldman, G. "Chickenpox vaccine: a cycle of disease. Appendix 3. Clinical descriptions of five different serious adverse affects that followed varicella vaccination." *Nexus New Times Magazine* (July-August 2007).

20. National Vaccine Information Center. "MedAlerts: access to the U.S. government's Vaccine Adverse Event Reporting System (VAERS)." www.medalerts.org

21. Roan, S. "Stubborn chickenpox fighting back." *The New Mexican* (April 28, 2007): D-2. Reprinted from *The Los Angeles Times*.

22. Goldman, G. "Universal varicella vaccination: efficacy trends and effect on herpes zoster." *International Journal of Toxicology* 2005;24:205-213.

23. Goldman, G. "International journal of toxicology release: chickenpox vaccine associated with shingles epidemic." *PRNewswire* (September 1, 2005).

24. Goldman, G. "Cost-benefit analysis of universal varicella vaccination in the U.S. taking into account the closely related herpes zoster epidemiology." *Vaccine* (May 9, 2005): 3349-3355.

25. Goldman, G. "Chickenpox vaccine associated with shingles epidemic." Press release: August 2005.

26. See Note 1.

27. Salzman, MB., et al. "Transmission of varicella-vaccine virus from a healthy 12-month-old child to his pregnant mother." *Journal of Pediatrics* (July 1997);131(1 Pt 1):151-54.

28. See Note 20.

29. See Note 13, p. 1277.

30. Halloran, ME., et al. "Theoretical epidemiologic and morbidity effects of routine varicella immunization of preschool children in the United States." *American Journal of Epidemiology* 1994;140:81-104.

31. National Foundation for Infectious Diseases. *What Parents Need to Know About Chickenpox* (informational pamphlet). Bethesda, MD.

32. New Yorkers for Vaccination Information and Choice. "What you should consider before taking the chickenpox vaccine (Varivax)." www.nyvic.org

33. Chaves, SA., et al. "Loss of vaccine-induced immunity to varicella over time." *New England Journal of Medicine* (March 15, 2007);356:1123-24.

34. See Notes 1 and 20.

35. Ibid.

36. Thinktwice Global Vaccine Institute. Unsolicited case report submitted by a concerned

parent. www.thinktwice.com

37. See Note 13, p. 1277.

38. See Note 20.

39. See Note 1.

40. Ibid.

41. Ibid.

42. Watson, BM., et al. "Modified chickenpox in children immunized with Oka-Merck varicella vaccine." *Pediatrics* 1993;91:17-22.

43. Naruse, H., et al. "Varicella infection complicated with meningitis after immunization." *Acta Paediatrica Japonica* 1993;35:345-47.

44. See Notes 13 and 20.

45. See Note 13, p. 1278.

46. See Note 36.

47. See Note 33.

48. See Note 1.

49. Ibid.

50. Ibid.

51. Close, J. *Kern Valley Sun* (Oct 20, 1999). www.kvsun.com

52. Barclay, L. "Guidelines updates for varicella prevention in children, teens, adults." *Medscape Medical News* (June 26, 2007). www.medscape.com

Hepatitis A

What is hepatitis A?
Hepatitis A is a contagious liver disease usually transmitted through contaminated food or water, or by coming into close contact with someone who is already infected. Symptoms may be similar to the flu, with low-grade fever, loss of appetite, fatigue and abdominal pain. Jaundice is possible. The disease is rarely as serious as other types of viral hepatitis.[1] Most people who are infected recover completely. There is no risk of long-term or chronic hepatitis A infection. Once you contract the disease and recover —typically in less than 2 months—you will not get it again.

Who is most at risk?
The groups at greatest risk of contracting hepatitis A are persons traveling to regions of the world with high rates of this disease, men who have sex with other men, illicit drug users, and persons with blood clotting disorders. Young children are *not* among the groups at greatest risk.[2]

The hepatitis A vaccine:
- Vaqta—Derived from hepatitis A virus grown in human MRC-5 diploid fibroblasts (originated from aborted human fetal tissue). Each dose also contains 225mcg of aluminum (450mcg per adult dose), sodium borate, sodium chloride, bovine albumin (cow blood proteins) and formaldehyde. Produced by Merck. Given in 2 doses.[3]
- Havrix—The hepatitis A virus is made in MRC-5 human diploid cells. Each dose also contains 250mcg of aluminum (500mcg per adult dose), polysorbate 20, residual MRC-5 cellular proteins, neomycin, and formaldehyde. Produced by GSK. Given in 2 doses.[4]
- Twinrix —contains both the hepatitis A and hepatitis B vaccines for persons 18 years of age or older.

Safety

The manufacturer lists several serious adverse reactions that were reported after hepatitis A vaccine was given. These include Guillain-Barré syndrome, thrombocytopenia, cerebellar ataxia, and encephalitis. Other serious adverse reactions following this vaccine have been reported as well, including anaphylaxis, brachial plexus neuropathy, transverse myelitis, encephalopathy, lymphadenopathy, meningitis, hepatitis, diabetes, and multiple sclerosis. Headache, upper respiratory infection, ear infection, menstruation disorder, myalgia, asthma, wheezing, allergic reactions, dermatitis, and diarrhea are also listed as commonly reported side effects.

The FDA and CDC also receive numerous reports confirming "neurologic, hematologic, and autoimmune syndromes" linked to this vaccine.[5-8]

Efficacy

According to the CDC, "the overall incidence of hepatitis A has declined in the United States over the past several decades primarily as a result of better hygienic and sanitary conditions."[9] According to the manufacturer, the duration of protection "is unknown at present." For example, in a 6-year follow-up study of children and adolescents who received 2 doses of the hepatitis A vaccine, researchers were only able to note "detectable" levels of anti-hepatitis A antibodies in test subjects—a measure far short of the "protective" levels sought.[10] Thus, immunity is most likely brief; additional booster shots may be recommended in the future.

Is the hepatitis A vaccine necessary?

Although children are not among the groups at greatest risk from this disease, authorities believe that "routine vaccination of children is the most effective way to reduce hepatitis A incidence nationwide."[11] Yet in 2004, *after* children under 5 years of age began receiving the hepatitis A vaccine, there was a 26 percent *increase* in the number of children under 5 years of age who contracted the disease: 231 cases in 2003 versus 291 cases in 2004.[12] In other words, children are being subjected to all of the potential hazards of this vaccine, with limited or questionable personal benefits, as part of an immunization strategy to protect high risk groups whose members are either difficult to reach or have rejected the shot.

Notes

1. Mayo Clinic Staff. "Hepatitis A." Mayo Clinic. www.MayoClinic.com (Sep 12, 2005).
2. Immunization Action Coalition. "Ask the experts: hepatitis A." www.immunize.org (Updated: June 2009).
3. Merck & Co., Inc. "(Hepatitis A Vaccine, Inactivated) Vaqta®." Product insert from the vaccine manufacturer. Issued: June 2006.
4. GlaxoSmithKline Biologicals. "Havrix® (Hepatitis A Vaccine, Inactivated)." Prescribing information from the vaccine manufacturer (December 2006).
5. CDC. "Prevention of hepatitis A through active or passive immunization: recommendations of the ACIP." *MMWR Weekly* (Oct. 1, 1999);48(RR12):23-24.
6. SmithKline Beecham Biologicals, unpublished data.
7. U.S. Department of Health and Human Services. "Vaccine Adverse Event Reporting System (VAERS)." www.hhs.gov
8. See Notes 3 and 4.
9. See Note 5, p. 14.
10. See Note 3.
11. See Note 5, p. 1.
12. CDC. *MMWR: Summary of Notifiable Diseases—U.S.*, 2003 (April 22, 2005);52(54); 2004 (June 16, 2006); 53(53).

Hepatitis B

What is hepatitis B?

Hepatitis B is a viral infection. Symptoms may be similar to the flu, including weakness, loss of appetite, nausea, vomiting, a low-grade fever, diarrhea, sore muscles and joint pain. A swollen liver and jaundice (yellowing of the skin and eyes) are possible as well. In some instances, individuals who contract this disease are carriers of the virus yet exhibit few or none of these symptoms. Acute hepatitis B usually runs its course within a few months. Most patients do not require hospital care and 95 percent recover completely; they will not contract the disease again. Long-term or chronic hepatitis B infections can be serious. Authorities estimate that about 20 percent of chronic cases eventually progress to liver damage, causing about 4,500 deaths annually.

How is hepatitis B contracted?

In the United States, about half of all new cases among adults occur through sexual transmission. The virus is spread through contact with the body fluids—blood, saliva and semen—of an infected person. People who inject illegal drugs account for another 15 percent of new cases, mainly by sharing needles with infected persons. It is also possible to contract hepatitis B by being stuck with a used needle, through improperly screened blood transfusions, or during birth when the virus passes from an infected mother to her baby.

Who is most at risk?

The groups at greatest risk of contracting hepatitis B are heterosexuals engaging in unprotected sex with multiple sex partners, prostitutes, sexually active homosexual men, intravenous drug users, healthcare and public safety workers exposed to infected body fluids, and household contacts of persons with chronic hepatitis B infection. Black Americans contract hepatitis B at higher rates than Asians and at rates 2 to 3 times greater than Whites. Infants born to infected mothers have a greater chance of acquiring this disease than babies born to non-infected mothers. *Children rarely develop this disease.* In the United States, less than one percent of all cases occur in persons less than 15 years of age.[1,2] The disease is even more uncommon in babies and toddlers. For example, in 2005 there were only 5 cases of hepatitis B in this age group.[3]

Persistent Exposure to Hepatitis B may Provide Benefits

The *American Journal of Epidemiology* published a study showing that healthcare workers increase their risk of contracting hepatitis B through frequency of contact with blood, but not through frequency of contact with patients. The authors of the study concluded that healthcare workers may become *passively immunized,* rather than infected, through continuous exposure to low levels of hepatitis B.[4]

The hepatitis B vaccine:

- Engerix-B—A "recombinant DNA" vaccine made by culturing genetically engineered yeast cells. Each dose contains sodium chloride, phosphate buffers, yeast protein, and 250mcg of aluminum (500mcg per adult dose). Produced by GSK. Given in 3 doses.[5]
- Recombivax HB—A recombinant vaccine "derived from hepatitis B surface antigen produced in yeast cells." Each dose contains a phosphate buffer, formaldehyde, plus 250mcg of aluminum (500mcg per adult dose). Produced by Merck. Given in 3 doses.[6]

Combination vaccines containing hepatitis B are available as well. These include Pediarix (DTaP/Polio/Hep B) and Twinrix (Hep A/B).

Safety

The clinical studies used to assess the safety of the current hepatitis B vaccine were comprised of just 147 healthy infants and children who were monitored for just 5 days after each shot. This is not a large enough sample nor long enough time period to determine true rates of adverse events. In fact, the manufacturer admits that "broad use of the vaccine could reveal adverse reactions not observed in clinical trials." Adult test subjects were monitored for only 5 days after each shot as well.[7]

The manufacturer lists several serious adverse reactions that have been reported after the hepatitis B vaccine was licensed and mass marketed. These include multiple sclerosis, transverse myelitis, arthritis, lupus, Guillain-Barré syndrome, thrombocytopenia (a serious blood clotting disorder), seizures, peripheral neuropathy, Bell's palsy, radiculopathy, encephalitis, Stevens-Johnson syndrome, eczema, alopecia (loss of hair), anaphylaxis, bronchial spasms, herpes zoster, tachycardia, optic neuritis, visual disturbances, and hearing disorders.[8] Although official fact sheets and other public endorsements of the hepatitis B vaccine minimize or deny serious reactions, numerous studies published in medical and scientific journals throughout the world, plus frequent reports filed with the FDA's Vaccine Adverse Event Reporting System (VAERS), confirm these and other afflictions following hepatitis B vaccination.[9,10]

Can the hepatitis B vaccine cause MULTIPLE SCLEROSIS?

Numerous studies have documented autoimmune and neurological disorders—including multiple sclerosis (MS)—after hepatitis B vaccination. For example, in 2004 *Neurology* published a study showing that hepatitis B vaccination is associated with a statistically significant elevated risk of multiple sclerosis.[11] In 2006, *Chinese Medical Journal* documented multiple sclerosis after hepatitis B vaccination.[12] In 2008, *Neurology* published two new studies showing statistically significant correlations between hepatitis B vaccination in children and the development of pediatric multiple sclerosis (central nervous system demyelination) more than three years later.[13,14]

Although many parents are unaware that the hepatitis B vaccine can lead to multiple sclerosis-like illnesses, some make the connection. For example, one mother wrote the following:

> *"My son was healthy until he got a hep B vaccine. Shortly after that he came down with the 'flu' and was then diagnosed with multiple sclerosis."*[15]
> **—Mother of a neurologically-damaged child**

Children are not the only ones susceptible to MS after receiving the hepatitis B vaccine. Here is one woman's description of her experience:

> *"Ever since I received the hepatitis B vaccine I have had weakness and heaviness in my legs, among other symptoms. I've seen several doctors and had many tests to determine what is wrong with me. I am in the category of multiple sclerosis-like symptoms."*[16]
> **—Adult victim of MS after receiving the hepatitis B vaccine**

Is the hepatitis B vaccine causing DIABETES?

The *New Zealand Medical Journal* published two papers linking the hepatitis B vaccine to epidemics of insulin-dependent diabetes mellitus (IDDM).[17,18] The lead author of the studies found that in the three years following a newly instituted national hepatitis B immunization campaign, there was a 60 percent increase in cases of IDDM. In fact...

"If we immunized every child after 8 weeks of life with the hepatitis B vaccine there may be an extra 4,000 to 5,000 cases of diabetes per year. On average, each case may cost $1 million in lost productivity and medical expenses. The estimated liability cost of the vaccine-induced diabetes is over $10 billion per year. The current cumulative liabilities to the U.S. government and to manufacturers could exceed $250 billion."[19]

—**J. Barthelow Classen, MD**

Additional hepatitis B vaccine safety issues:

Several studies throughout the world have documented both acute and chronic arthritis after hepatitis B vaccination.[20-31] Numerous studies have also documented skin, liver, kidney, vision, hearing, and blood disorders after hepatitis B vaccination.[32-87] For example, recent studies in *The Lancet,* the *Scandinavian Journal of Infectious Diseases,* the *Archives of Disease in Childhood*, and the *European Journal of Pediatrics* all confirmed that thrombocytopenia—a serious disease causing bleeding, bruising and clotting problems—can occur after hepatitis B vaccination.[88]

In September 2009, *NeuroToxicology* published a study in which some monkeys received a mercury-based hepatitis B vaccine shortly after birth while others received a placebo. The vaccinated monkeys developed significant delays in critical survival reflexes and sensorimotor skills, such as sucking on a nipple. Infants of lower birth weight and gestational age were at even greater risk.[89]

The case reports on the following page were taken directly from the FDA's Vaccine Adverse Event Reporting System (VAERS).[90] They are a small sample of the potential side effects linked to the hepatitis B vaccine.

Efficacy

Hepatitis B vaccine efficacy is defined by injecting subjects with the shot then measuring the number of anti-hepatitis B antibodies that are produced in the blood. These antibodies must meet or exceed a predetermined level established by researchers, a basis presumed to provide protective benefits. Scientists call this "seroprotection." According to this definition, the vaccine is considered "highly immunogenic" when antibody levels are measured shortly after the last dose of the 3-dose vaccine regimen is administered. However, according to the vaccine manufacturer, "the duration of the protective effect in healthy vaccinees is unknown."[91] In fact, follow-up studies just a few years later show that approximately half of all vaccinated people fail to maintain protective antibody levels.

Hepatitis B Vaccine: VAERS Case Reports

▸160271: A 4-month-old boy received the hepatitis B vaccine, developed acute diarrhea, went into a coma, and died that evening.

▸49808: A 4-month-old girl received the hepatitis B shot, developed a bleeding disorder, encephalitis, and abnormal liver function. She died 3 days later.

▸107120: A 5-month-old boy received the hepatitis B vaccine, developed a fever, and died of sudden infant death syndrome the following day.

▸76188: A 6-month-old girl received the hepatitis B vaccine, developed diarrhea, bleeding lesions, Stevens-Johnson syndrome, and died 2 days later.

▸179608: A 6-month-old girl received the hepatitis B vaccine and developed "severe neurological sequelae" 8 hours later. She was hospitalized with apnea, convulsions, cerebral edema, fontanelle bulging, and psychomotor retardation.

▸49035: A 7-month-old girl received the hepatitis B vaccine, developed a cerebral hemorrhage and died 4 days later.

▸114934: A 7-month-old boy received the hepatitis B shot, slept 16 hours, then had delayed psychomotor development and mental retardation.

▸160183: A 9-month-old baby received the hepatitis B vaccine (Engerix-B) and died 18 hours later.

▸180302: A 10-month-old girl received the hepatitis B shot, developed a bacterial infection, bronchiolitis, went into a coma, and died the next day.

▸74126: A 10-month-old girl received the hepatitis B vaccine, developed liver cancer one month later, and died from her condition.

▸173745: A 1½-year-old girl received the hepatitis B vaccine and later that evening was found dead with profuse bleeding from her mouth and nose.

▸212894: A 3-year-old girl received the hepatitis B vaccine and developed juvenile onset diabetes mellitus 25 days later.

For example, the *New England Journal of Medicine* showed that after just five years hepatitis B antibody levels declined sharply or no longer existed in 42 percent of the vaccine recipients. In addition, 34 of the 773 subjects (4.4 percent!) became infected with the virus.[92,93] In 2005, the *Pediatric Infectious Disease Journal* published data confirming that babies who had received the standard 3-dose series of hepatitis B vaccine quickly lost protective antibodies. Just 47 percent of the children showed adequate antibody levels by 2 years of age. By 5 years of age, 81 percent of the children failed to maintain protective antibody levels.[94] In 2009, the *Canadian Medical Association* acknowledged that "the controversy surrounding booster injections stems in part from the rapid drop in antibodies after completion of the primary series of injections."[95] The medical literature contains corroborating data documenting vaccine failures.[96,97]

On the following page are firsthand accounts by the parents of children who developed serious ailments after receiving the hepatitis B vaccine.[98]

Case Reports by Parents

▸ *"After our son was born, they injected him with hepatitis B vaccine. He immediately suffered a seven minute seizure. Now our son has Sensory Integration Dysfunction."*

▸ *"Our daughter was born healthy but received the hepatitis B vaccine, and at three days old she started having seizures. After a week in the local children's hospital, it was discovered that she had suffered a stroke."*

▸ *"My grandson had a hepatitis B vaccine at two days old. He was sent home from the hospital and returned later in the afternoon to the emergency room because he wasn't breathing properly. A few days later he was having seizures. One month later he again had the vaccination and ended up at the ER again with the same problem. Doctors tell us that it is not because of the vaccination, however I am very concerned about letting him have the third shot."*

▸ *"My little boy was injured by a hepatitis B vaccine given to him when he was only three days old. The adverse reaction was so severe that he had an aneurysm rupture in his brain. He has many complications and is severely brain damaged. His life was taken from him. He has seizure disorder, epilepsy, cortical blindness, a feeding tube, and is immobile."*

▸ *"My son was healthy until five days after he received his hepatitis B vaccination. He has since been chronically ill for two years."*

▸ *"Our son was born six weeks premature and reacted badly to his shots. After the first, he cried and had a head circumference growth of 4.25cm in four days. After the second shot he stopped breathing. He had brain swelling, bleeding in the brain and behind the eyes. He has multiple problems from this. I did not know about vaccine damage before it happened to us."*

▸ *"Our daughter received a hepatitis B vaccine. She was then hospitalized with a fever and thrombocytopenia (a serious blood disorder)."*

▸ *"I am a mother of three boys, but the problem with my family is, we lost our dear baby when he was almost two months old. He passed away after receiving just one shot of the hepatitis B vaccine!"*

▸ *"My 5-year-old daughter slumped to the floor after receiving her second dose of the hepatitis B vaccine. That is when the nurse gave us a side effects sheet and was telling me when to bring her back for another shot."*

▸ *"Our 6-year-old son became ill after his first dose of hepatitis B vaccine. He had a fever of 103 degrees for five days. After his second dose he had a fever that did not go away. Three months later he was diagnosed with rheumatic fever. One month later his blood counts dropped and he was rediagnosed with A.L.L. leukemia."*

Is the hepatitis B vaccine necessary?

In 1991, the CDC recommended that all infants receive the hepatitis B vaccine. Today, states mandate this shot. Yet, surveys in medical journals indicate that up to 87 percent of pediatricians and family practitioners do not believe this vaccine is needed by their newborn patients.[99,100] However, "because a vaccination strategy limited to high-risk individuals has failed,"[101] and since children are "more accessible,"[102] they are now compelled to receive the three-shot series beginning at birth. In other words, because high-risk groups are difficult to reach or have rejected this vaccine, authorities are targeting babies—even though babies are not likely to contract this disease. *Babies are being subjected to all of the risks of this vaccine without the expected benefit.* Due to waning efficacy or partial immunity, older children are compelled to receive booster doses as well. In addition, some companies are demanding hepatitis B shots for adults as a condition of employment. Grown-ups must carefully weigh the risks and benefits. Parents should know that each state permits them to legally exempt their children from "mandatory" shots.

Notes

1. Alter, MJ., et al. "The changing epidemiology of hepatitis B in the United States." *Journal of the American Medical Association* 1990;263:1218-1222.

2. CDC. *MMWR, Morbidity and Mortality Weekly Report: Summary of Notifiable Diseases—United States, 2003* (April 22, 2005);Vol. 52, No. 54.

3. CDC. *MMWR: Summary of Notifiable Diseases—United States, 2003* (April 22, 2005);Vol. 52, No. 54 and *2005* (March 30, 2007);54(53): Table 3.

4. Dienstag, JL., et al. "Occupational exposure to hepatitis B virus in hospital personnel: infection or immunization?" *Amer J of Epidemiology* 1982;115(1):26-39.

5. GlaxoSmithKline Biologicals. "Engerix-B [Hepatitis B Vaccine (Recombinant)]." Product insert from the vaccine manufacturer (2009).

6. Merck & Co., Inc. "Recombivax HB Hepatitis B Vaccine (Recombinant)." Product insert from the vaccine manufacturer (Issued: December 2007).

7. Ibid.

8. See Notes 5 and 6.

9. See Notes 11-14, 17-18, and 20-87.

10. National Vaccine Information Center. "MedAlerts: access to the U.S. government's Vaccine Adverse Event Reporting System (VAERS)." www.medalerts.org

11. Hernán, MA., et al. "Recombinant hepatitis B vaccine and the risk of multiple sclerosis: a prospective study." *Neurology* 2004;63:838-842.

12. Terney, D., et al. "Multiple sclerosis after hepatitis B vaccination in a 16-year-old patient." *Chinese Medical Journal* 2006;119(1):77-79.

13. Yann, M., et al. "Hepatitis B vaccine and the risk of CNS inflammatory demyelination in childhood." *Neurology* (October 8, 2008). [published online]

14. Ness, JM., et al. "Hepatitis vaccines and pediatric multiple sclerosis. Does timing or type matter?" *Neurology* (December 17, 2008). [published online]

15. Thinktwice Global Vaccine Institute. Unsolicited case reports submitted by concerned parents. www.thinktwice.com

16. Ibid.

17. Classen, John Barthelow. "Childhood immunisation and diabetes mellitus," *New Zealand Medical Journal* (May 24, 1996):195.

18. Classen, John Barthelow. "The diabetes epidemic and the hepatitis B vaccine." *New Zealand Medical Journal* (May 24, 1996):366.

19. Classen, J. Barthelow. "Hepatitis B vaccine: helping or hurting public health?" Congressional Testimony. *Subcommittee on Criminal Justice, Drug Policy and Human Resources; Committee on Govt. Reform* (Wash., DC: May 18, 1999).

20. Rogerston, SJ., et al. "Hepatitis B vaccine associated with erythema nodosum and polyarthritis." *British Medical Journal* 1990;301:345.

21. Hachulla, E., et al. "Reactive arthritis after hepatitis B vaccination." *Journal of Rheumatology* 1990; 17:1250-1251.

22. Vautier, G., et al. "Acute sero-positive rheumatoid arthritis occurring after hepatitis vaccination." *Br J Rheumatol* (October 1994);33(10):991.

23. Hassan, W., et al. "Reiter's syndrome and reactive arthritis in health care workers after vaccination." *British Medical Journal* (July 9, 1994);309(6967):94.

24. Birley, HD., et al. "Hepatitis B immunisation and reactive arthritis." *BMJ* 1994 Dec;309(6967):1514.

25. Aherne, P., et al. "Psoriatic arthropathy." *Irish Med J* (Mar-April, 1995); 88(2):72.

26. Harrison, BJ., et al. "Patients who develop inflammatory polyarthritis (IP) after immunization are clinically indistinguishable from other patients with IP." *Br J Rheumatol* (March 1997);36(3):366-9.

27. Bracci, M., et al. "Polyarthritis associated with hepatitis B vaccination." *British J Rheumatol* (February 1997);36(2):300-1.

28. Pope, JE., et al. "The development of rheumatoid arthritis after recombinant hepatitis B vaccination." *J Rheumatol* (September 1998);25(9):1687-93.

29. Grasland, A., et al. "Adult-onset Still's disease after hepatitis A and B vaccination?" *Rev Med Interne* (February 1998);19(2):134-6.

30. Maillefert, JF., et al. "Rheumatic disorders developed after hepatitis B vaccination." *Rheumatol* (Oxford), (October 1999);38(10):978-83.

31. Toussirot, E., et al. "Sjogren's syndrome occurring after hepatitis B vaccination." *Arthritis Rheuma* (September 2000);43(9):2139-40.

32. Goolsby, PL. "Erythema nodosum after Recombivax HB hepatitis B vaccine." *N Engl J Med* (October 1989);321:1198-9.

33. Castresana-Isla, CJ., et al. "Erythema nodosum and Takayasu's arteritis after immunization with plasma derived hepatitis B vaccine." *J Rheum* (Aug 1993);20(8):1417-8.

34. Trevisan, G., et al. "Lichen ruber planus following HBV vaccination." *Acta Dermato-Venereologica* (February 1993);73(1):73.

35. Aubin, F., et al. "Lichen planus following hepatitis B vaccination." *Archives of Dermatology* (October 1994);130(10):1329-30.

36. Di Lernia, V., et al. "Bisighini G. Erythema multiforme following hepatitis B vaccine." *Ped Derma* (December 1994);11(4):363-4.

37. Saywell, CA., et al. "Kossard S. Lichenoid reaction to hepatitis B vaccination." *Australasian J Derm* (August 1997);38(3):152-4.

38. Ferrando, MF., et al. "Lichen planus following hepatitis B vaccination." *Br J Dermatol* (Aug 1998);139(2):350.

39. Barbaud, A., et al. "Allergic mechanisms and urticaria/angioedema after hepatitis B immunization." *Br J Dermatol* (November 1998);139(5):925-6.

40. Schupp, P., et al. "Lichen planus following hepatitis B vaccination." *International Journal of Dermatology* (October 1999);38(10):799-800.

41. Loche, F., et al. "Erythema multiforme associated with hepatitis B immunization." *Clin Exp Dermatol* (March 2000);25(2):167-8.

42. Al-Khenaizan, S. "Lichen planus occurring after hepatitis B vaccination: a new case." *J Am Acad Dermatol* (October 2001);45(4):614-5.

43. Ranieri, VM., et al. "Liver inflammation and acute respiratory distress syndrome in a patient receiving hepatitis B vaccine: a possible relationship?" *Intensive Care Medicine* (January 1997);23(1):119-21.

44. Islek, I., et al. "Nephrotic syndrome following hepatitis B vaccination." *Pediatr Nephrol* (Jan 2000);14:89-90.

45. Fried, M., et al. "Uveitis after hepatitis B vaccination." *The Lancet* (Sep 12, 1987):631-2.

46. Brezin, A, et al. "Visual loss and eosinophilia after recombinant hepatitis B vaccine." *The Lancet* (August 28, 1993);342(8870):563-4.

47. Achiron, LR, et al. "Postinfectious hepatitis B optic neuritis." *Optom Vis Sci* 1994; 71:53-6.

48. Brezin, AP, et al. "Acute posterior multifocal placoid pigment epitheliopathy after hepatitis B vaccine." *Arch Ophthalmol* (March 1995);113(3):297-300.

49. Devin, F., et al. "Occlusion of central retinal vein after hepatitis B vaccination." *Lancet* (June 1996); 347(9015):1626.

50. Baglivo, E, et al. "Multiple evanescent white dot syndrome after hepatitis B vaccine." *Am J Ophthalmol* (September 1996);122(3):431-2.

51. Berkman, N., et al. "Bilateral neuro-papillitis after hepatitis B vaccination." *Presse Med* (September 28, 1996);25(28):1301. [French.]

52. Bonfils, P., et al. "Fluctuant perception hearing loss after hepatitis B vaccine." *Ann Otolaryngol Chir Cervicofac* 1996;113(6):359-61. [French.]

53. Granel, B, et al. "Occlusion of the central retinal vein after vaccination against viral hepatitis B with recombinant vaccines." *Presse Med* (Feb 1, 1997);26(2):62-5. [French.]

54. Albitar, S., et al. "Bilateral retrobulbar optic neuritis with hepatitis B vaccination." *Nephrol Dial Transplant* (October 1997);12(10):2169-70.

55. Arya, SC. "Ophthalmic complications of vaccines against hepatitis B virus." *Int Ophth* 1997;21(3):177-8.

56. Bourges, JL., et al. "Multifocal placoid epitheliopathy and anti-hepatitis B vaccination." *J Fr Ophtalmol* (November 1998);21(9):696-700. [French.]

57. Cockwell, P., et al. "Vasculitis related to hepatitis B vaccine." *BMJ* (Dec 1, 1990); 301(6763):1281.

58. Allen, MB., et al. "Pulmonary and cutaneous vasculitis following hepatitis B vaccination." *Thorax* (May 1993);48(5):580-1.

59. Nagafuchi, S., et al. "Eosinophilia after intradermal hepatitis B vaccination." *The Lancet* 1993;342:998.

60. Poullin, P., et al. "Thrombocytopenic purpura after recombinant hepatitis B vaccine." *The Lancet* (November 1994);344(8932):1293.

61. Meyboom, RH., et al. "Thrombocytopenia reported in association with hepatitis B and A vaccines." *The Lancet* (June 1995);345(8965):1638.

62. Neau, D., et al. "Immune thrombocytopenic purpura after recombinant hepatitis B vaccine: retrospective study of seven cases." *Scan J. Infect Dis* 1998;30(2):115-8.

63. Ronchi, F., et al. "Thrombocytopenic purpura as adverse reaction to recombinant hepatitis B vaccine." *Arch Dis Child* (March 1998);78(3):273-4.

64. Muller, A., et al. "Thrombocytopenic purpura: adverse reaction to a combined immunisation (recombinant hepatitis B and measles-mumps-rubella-vaccine) and after therapy with Co-trimoxazole." *Eur J Pediatr* (December 1999);158 Suppl 3:S209-10.

65. Le Hello, C., et al. "Suspected hepatitis B vaccination related vasculitis." *Journal of Rheumatology* (January 1999);26(1):191-4.

66. Rabaud, C., et al "First case of erythermalgia related to hepatitis B vaccination." *Journal of Rheumatology* (January 1999);26(1):233-4.

67. De Keyser, F., et al. "Immune-mediated pathology following hepatitis B vaccination. Two cases of polyarteritis nodosa and one case of pityriasis rosea-like drug eruption." *Clin Exp Rheumatol* (Jan-Feb 2000);18(1):81-5.

68. Viallard, JF., et al. "Severe pancytopenia triggered by recombinant hepatitis B vaccine." *Br J Haematol* (July 2000);110(1):230-3.

69. Zaas, A., et al. "Large artery vasculitis following recombinant hepatitis B vaccination. 2 cases." *J Rheumatol* (May 2001);28(5):1116-20.

70. Conesa, V., et al. "Thrombocytopenic purpura after recombinant hepatitis B vaccine: a rare association." *Haematologica* (March 2001);86(3):E09. [Italian.]

71. Herroelen, L., et al. "Central nervous system demyelination after immunization

with recombinant hepatitis B vaccine." *Lancet* (Nov. 9, 1991);338(8776):1174-75.

72. Tudela, P., et al. "Systemic lupus erythematosus and vaccination against hepatitis B." *Nephron* 1992 62(2):236.

73. Martinez, E., et al. "Evan's syndrome triggered by recombinant hepatitis B vaccine." *Clin Infect Dis.* 1992;15:1051.

74. Ganry, O., et al. "Peripheral facial paralysis following vaccination against hepatitis B. Apropos of a case." *Therapie* 1992;47:437-438.

75. Trevisani, F., et al. "Transverse myelitis following hepatitis B vaccination." *Journal of Hepatology* (September 1993);19(2):317-8.

76. Mamoux, V., et al. "Lupus erthymatosus disseminatus and vaccination against hepatitis B virus." *Arch Pediatr* 1994;1:307-309.

77. Kaplanski, G., et al. "Central nervous system demyelination after vaccination against hepatitis B...." *J Neurol Neurosurg Psychiatry* (June 1995);58(6):758-9.

78. Guiserix, J. "Systemic lupus erythematosus following hepatitis B vaccine." *Nephron* 1996;74(2):441.

79. Manna, R., et al. "Leukoencephalitis after recombinant hepatitis B vaccine." *Journal of Hepatology* (June 1996);24(6):764-5.

80. Mathieu, E., et al. "Cryoglobulinemia after hepatitis B vaccination." *New England J Med* (Aug 1996); 335(5):335.

81. Cohen, AD., et al. "Vaccine-induced autoimmunity." *J Autoimmunity* (Dec 1996); 9(6):699-703.

82. Kakar, A., et al. "Guillain Barre syndrome associated with hepatitis B vaccination." *Indian J Ped* (Sept-Oct 1997);64(5):710-2.

83. Wise, RP., et al. "Hair loss after routine immunizations." *JAMA* (Oct 8, 1997):1176-8.

84. Flemmer, M., et al. "The bald truth." *Am J Gastroenterol* (April 1999); 94(4):1104.

85. Creange, A., et al. "Lumbosacral acute demyelinating polyneuropathy following hepatitis B vaccination." *Autoimmunity* 1999;30:143-6.

86. Tourbah, A., et al. "Encephalitis after hepatitis B vaccination: recurrent disseminated encephalitis or MS?" *Neurology* (July 22, 1999);53(2):396-401.

87. Sinsawaiwong, S., et al. "Guillain-Barré syndrome following recombinant hepatitis B vaccine and literature review." *J Med Assoc Thai.* (Sept 2000); 83(9):1124-6.

88. See Notes 60-64.

89. Hewitson L,, et al. "Delayed acquisition of neonatal reflexes in newborn primates receiving a thimerosal-containing hepatitis B vaccine: influence of gestational age and birth weight. *Neurotoxicology* (October 2, 2009).

90. See Note 10.

91. See Notes 5 and 6.

92. Hadler, SC., et al. "Long-term immunogenicity and efficacy of hepatitis B vaccine in homosexual men." *New England Journal of Medicine* (July 24, 1986); Vol. 315:209-214.

93. Stevens, CE., et al. "Prospects for control of hepatitis B virus infection: implications of childhood vaccination and long-term protection." *Pediatrics* 1992;90:170-173.

94. Dentinger, CM., et al. "Persistence of antibody to hepatitia B and protection from disease among Alaska Natives immunized at birth." *Ped Infect Disease J* 2005;24(9):786-92.

95. Mackie, CO., et al. "Hepatitis B immunization strategies: timing is everything." *Canadian Medical Association Journal* (January 20, 2009).

96. Ballinger, AB., et al. "Severe acute hepatitis B infection after vaccination." *Lancet* 1994;344:1292-1293

97. Goffin, E., et al. "Acute hepatitis B infection after vaccination." *Lancet* 1995;345:263.

98. See Note 15.

99. Freed, GL., et al. "Reactions of pediatricians to a new CDC recommendation for universal immunization of infants with hepatitis B vaccine." *Pediatrics* 1993;91:699-702.

100. Freed, GL., et al. "Family physician acceptance of universal hepatitis B immunization of infants." *Journal of Family Practice* 1993;36:153-157.

101. See Notes 5 and 6.

102. Schaffner, W., et al. "Hepatitis B immunization strategies: expanding the target." *Annals of Internal Medicine* (February 15, 1993);118(4):308.

Haemophilus Influenzae Type B (Hib)

What is Haemophilus influenzae type b?

Haemophilus influenzae type b, or Hib (no relation to the flu), is a serious bacterial infection spread through sneezing, coughing, and secretions from an infected person. Meningitis (inflammation of the membranes surrounding the brain and spinal cord) occurs in about half of the cases. Around 20 percent of all Hib infections cause hearing loss, neurological problems, or pneumonia. Nearly 15 percent of cases result in epiglottitis (inflammation of the throat). The case-fatality rate is about four percent. Treatment mainly consists of intravenously administered antibiotics. Other medical interventions may also be required.

How prevalent is Hib?

Hib infections were very uncommon in the first half of the 20th century. However, Hib rates jumped by 400 percent between 1946 and 1986[1,2] (see sidebar). During the 1970s and 1980s, there were an estimated 16,000 to 20,000 Hib infections per year in the United States. Rates tumbled during the 1990s and 2000s. Today, there are less than 100 cases per year.

Who is most susceptible to Hib?

Sixty percent of all Hib cases occur in children less than 12 months of age; 90 percent occur in children less than five years of age. In addition, the following groups have an increased risk of contracting Hib: Blacks, Hispanics and Native Americans; children living in crowded conditions or placed in daycare; people with weakened immune systems.

The Hib vaccine:

Hib Vaccines were first licensed in the late 1980s and early 1990s. Three Hib "conjugate" vaccines (and several combination shots containing Hib) are currently available. The CDC recommends several doses for infants and young children.

- ActHIB—Contains polysaccharides from "Hib strain 1482 grown in a semi-synthetic medium, covalently bound to tetanus toxoid." Also contains sodium chloride, sucrose, and formalin (formaldehyde and methanol). Produced by Sanofi Pasteur. Given in 4 doses.[3]
- HibTITER—Contains polysaccharides from the Hib "Eagan" strain conjugated with the diphtheria toxoid. Also contains sodium chloride. Produced by Wyeth. Given in 4 doses.[4]

**What Caused Hib Rates to Dramatically Increase
During the Second Half of the 20th Century?**

One theory is that the overuse of antibiotics during the first part of the 20th century caused Hib bacteria to mutate and become more resistant. Another possibility is that the DPT vaccine—introduced in 1936 and put into general use in the 1940s—was responsible for the new bacterial infections. Several studies confirm that vaccinations can "provoke" or cause new diseases. For example, the *Journal of Infectious Diseases* published a study confirming "disease accentuation after immunization."[5] In addition, *The Lancet* published data showing that when Sweden introduced a new DPT vaccine, the number of invasive bacterial infections statistically increased.[6] And when Japan stopped vaccinating babies with DPT, bacterial meningitis rates declined.[7,8]

- PedvaxHIB—Contains polysaccharides from the Hib "Ross" strain covalently bound to "the B11 strain of *Neisseria meningitidis* serogroup B." Also contains sodium chloride and 225mcg of aluminum. Produced by Merck. Given in 3 doses.[9]

Combination vaccines containing Hib include: TriHIBit (Hib/DTaP); Pentacel (Hib/DTaP/Polio); and Comvax (Hib/Hepatitis B).

Safety

Hib vaccines are often administered simultaneously with other vaccines. Thus, when a child experiences an adverse reaction to the shot, it is often difficult to ascertain which component of the vaccine (or of the several simultaneously administered vaccines) is responsible. Nevertheless, the medical literature contains ample documentation confirming possible correlations between the Hib vaccine and serious ailments, including: Guillain-Barré syndrome, insulin-dependent diabetes mellitus, early onset Hib disease, transverse myelitis (paralysis of the spinal cord), aseptic meningitis, invasive pneumococcal disease, upper respiratory infection, otitis media (ear infection), thrombocytopenia (a decrease in blood platelets leading to internal bleeding), erythema multiforme (allergic skin disease), fever, rash, hives, vomiting, diarrhea, high-pitched crying, seizures, convulsions, and sudden infant death syndrome.[10-16]

Quick Facts About Hib

♦ **Breastfed babies are less likely to contract Hib.** Nursing was found to have a protective effect against Hib infections.[17,18]

♦ **Hib does not spread easily.** According to the CDC, "the contagious potential of invasive Hib disease is considered to be limited."[19]

♦ **Some people are naturally immune to Hib.** Thirty percent of all healthy people are carriers of the microorganism that "causes" Hib, yet never show symptoms of the disease.[20]

Can the Hib vaccine cause DIABETES?

Sharp increases of insulin-dependent diabetes mellitus (type 1 diabetes) have been recorded in the U.S., England, and other countries following mass immunization campaigns with the Hib vaccine.[21,22] Data published in the *British Medical Journal* and *Autoimmunity* divided more than 200,000 Finnish children into three groups.[23-25] The first group received NO doses of the Hib vaccine. The second group received one dose of the Hib vaccine (at 24 months of age). The third group received four doses of the Hib vaccine (at 3, 4, 6, and 18 months of age).

Results: At ages 7 and 10, the total number of cases of type 1 diabetes in all three groups was tallied. At age 7, there were 54 more cases per 100,000 children in the group that received four doses of the Hib vaccine when compared to the group that received no doses—*a 26 percent increase!* At age 10, there were 58 more cases per 100,000 children in the group that received four doses of the Hib vaccine when compared to the group that received no doses.[26] Based on an annual birth rate of about 4 million children, in the United States alone this translates into 2,300 additional —and avoidable—cases of diabetes every year.[27] (Each case of insulin-dependent diabetes is estimated to cost more than $1 million in medical costs and lost productivity.)[28] By contrast, the Hib vaccine is expected to prevent a much smaller number of severe disabilities.[29] According to the lead author of this landmark study...

"The increased risk of diabetes in the vaccinated group exceeds the expected decreased risk of complications of Hib meningitis.... The potential risk of the vaccine exceeds the potential benefit."[30,31]
—J. Barthelow Classen, MD, lead author of a landmark study

Although many parents are unaware that the Hib vaccine can lead to diabetes, some make the connection. For example, one mother wrote the following:

> *"I have a son who was diagnosed with diabetes six months after his first Hib shot. Two of his friends were also diagnosed six months after their first Hib shot. There is no history of diabetes in any of these families."*[32]
> —**Mother of a Hib-vaccinated child**

The case reports on the following page were taken directly from the FDA's Vaccine Adverse Event Reporting System (VAERS).[33] They are a small sample of the potential side effects linked to the Hib vaccine.

Efficacy

Children are at risk of contracting Hib disease following their Hib vaccinations. For example, doctors have been warned by the CDC that cases of Hib may occur after vaccination, "prior to the onset of the protective effects of the vaccine."[34] This same warning is published by all three of the Hib vaccine manufacturers in their product inserts.[35] Other research warns of "increased susceptibility" to the disease during the first seven days after vaccination.[36] The American Academy of Pediatrics has warned doctors to warn parents to look for signs of the disease in their children following vaccination.[37] In fact, several studies found that Hib-vaccinated children are 2 to 6 times more likely than non-Hib-vaccinated children to contract Hib disease during the first week following vaccination.[38-42]

Additional research has confirmed that antibody levels *decline* rather than increase immediately following Hib vaccinations[43,44] —even with the newer conjugated Hib vaccines[45] —placing the child at *greater* risk for invasive disease. From 1998 to 2000, 32 percent of all children aged 6 months to 5 years with confirmed Hib disease had received three or more doses of Hib vaccine, including many who had received a booster dose 14 or more days before onset of their illness.[46]

Minorities: Although the evidence suggests that minority children are at greater risk of contracting Hib, a study published in the *New England Journal of Medicine* found the conjugated Hib vaccine to be ineffective at preventing Hib disease among a group of minority children.[47]

Hib Vaccine: VAERS Case Reports

▸301258: A 2-month-old boy developed thrombocytopenic purpura—internal bleeding—with "mass petechia in both extremities, and scattered petechia in face and trunks," 1 day after receiving a Hib vaccine.

▸189675: A 4-month-old girl received the Hib vaccine and died 2 days later.

▸176214: A 4-month-old boy died 3 days after receiving a Hib vaccine.

▸268399: A 4-month-old girl received the Hib vaccine and 5 hours later developed a fever and twitching. She was taken to the hospital where her heartbeat was recorded at 251 beats per minute and she became comatose.

▸57458: A 4-month-old girl received a series of Hib shots and developed Hib bacteremia, lymphadenopathy, and arthritis.

▸27509: A 4-month-old boy received the Hib vaccine and died the next day.

▸206193: Two days after receiving the Hib vaccine, a 4-month-old girl developed a fever, rash and seizures, with grimacing and "mouth smacking." She was transferred to two different hospitals.

▸312543: A 5-month-old girl received the Hib vaccine and went into respiratory arrest 2 days later. The cause of death was "undetermined."

▸44458: A 5-month-old girl received the Hib vaccine and 5 days later developed a fever, rash, life-threatening bacteremia and pneumonia.

▸337637: A 6-month-old boy developed a stroke 12 hours after receiving a Hib vaccine. Other symptoms were facial palsy, gaze palsy, brain edema and convulsions.

▸115531: A 6-month-old girl received the Hib vaccine, contracted meningitis, and died.

▸64420: A 10-month-old girl received the Hib vaccine, developed a respiratory disorder the following day, went into a stupor and became unconscious.

▸51401: A 10-month-old girl received the Hib vaccine and was hospitalized for Hib bacteremia 4 months later.

▸304028: A 1-year-old girl received a series of Hib shots and was hospitalized with epiglottitis—a condition linked with Hib infection—a few months later.

▸85470: A 13-month-old girl received the Hib vaccine and was admitted to the hospital with Hib meningitis.

▸111214: Within 18 hours of receiving the Hib vaccine, a 1½-year-old girl developed blood poisoning and starting hemorrhaging. She died 5 hours later.

▸106394: A 1½-year-old boy received a Hib shot and died of Hib meningitis.

▸59280: A 17-month-old boy received the Hib vaccine, developed life-threatening meningitis and was hospitalized.

▸56750: A 20-month-old girl received the Hib vaccine and developed Hib meningitis with septicemia 5 months later.

▸345253: A 16-month-old boy received the Hib vaccine, developed a high fever, vomiting, increased heart rate, and convulsions a few hours later.

▸339492: An 8-month-old boy developed thrombocytopenic purpura—a serious bleeding disorder—4 days after receiving a Hib vaccine.

Notes

1. Smith, E., et al. "Changing incidence of haemophilus influenzae meningitis." *Pediatrics* 1972;50(5):723-727.

2. Fisher, BL. *The Consumer's Guide to Childhood Vaccines.* (Vienna, VA: NVIC, 1997):21.

3. Sanofi Pasteur. "Haemophilus b Conjugate Vaccine (Tetanus Toxoid Conjugate) ActHIB." Product insert from the vaccine manufacturer (December 2005).

4. Wyeth Pharmaceuticals, Inc. "Haemophilus b Conjugate Vaccine (Diphtheria CRM$_{197}$ Protein Conjugate) HibTITER." Product insert from the vaccine manufacturer (Revised: January 2007).

5. Craighead, J E. "Report of a workshop: disease accentuation after immunization with inactivated microbial vaccines." *J of Infectious Diseases* 1975;1312(6):749-54.

6. Sutter, R., et al. "Attributable risk of DTP injection in provoking paralytic poliomyelitis during a large outbreak in Oman." *Journal of Infectious Diseases* 1992;165:444-449.

7. Kimura, M., et al. "Acellular pertussis vaccines and fatal infections." *The Lancet* (April 16, 1988):881-882.

8. Scheibner, V. *Vaccination: 100 Years of Orthodox Research.* (Blackheath, Australia: Scheibner Publications, 1993):133.

9. Merck & Co., Inc. "Liquid PedvaxHIB [Haemophilus b Conjugate Vaccine (Meningococcal Protein Conjugate)]" Product insert from the vaccine manufacturer (Issued: Jan 2001).

10. Institute of Medicine. *Adverse Events Associated with Childhood Vaccines: Evidence Bearing on Causality.* Wash., DC: National Academy Press, 1994.

11. Gervaix, M., et al. "Guillain-Barre syndrome following immunization with Haemophilus influenzae type b conjugate vaccine." *European Journal of Pediatrics* 1993;152:613-14.

12. D'Cruz, OF., et al. "Acute inflammatory demyelinating polyradiculoneuropathy (Guillain-Barre syndrome) after immunization with Haemophilus influenzae type b conjugate vaccine." *J of Pediatrics* 1989;115:743-46.

13. Vadheim, CM., et al. "Effectiveness and safety of an Haemophilus influenzae type b conjugate vaccine (PRP-T) in young infants." *Pediatrics* 1993;92:272-79.

14. Ward, J., et al. "Efficacy of a Haemophilus influenzae type b conjugate vaccine in Alaska native infants." *New England J of Med* 1990;323(2):1393-1401.

14. Milstien, JB., et al. "Adverse reactions reported following Haemophilus influenzae type b vaccine: an analysis after one year of marketing." *Pediatrics* 1987;80:270-74.

15. U.S. Department of Health and Human Services. "Vaccine Adverse Event Reporting System (VAERS)." www.hhs.gov

16. See Notes 3, 4, 9-15 and 24-26.

17. Harrison, LH., et al. "Haemophilus influenzae type b polysaccharide vaccine: an efficacy study." *Pediatrics* 1989; 84:255-61.

18. Istre, GR., et al. "Risk factors for primary invasive Haemophilus influenzae disease: increased risk from day-care attendance and school-aged household members." *Journal of Pediatrics* 1985;106:190-95.

19. CDC. "Haemophilus Influenzae Type b" in *The Pink Book, Epidemiology and Prevention of Vaccine Preventable Diseases,* 11th edition (May 2009):75. www.cdc.gov/vaccines/pubs/pinkbook

20. Mosby's Medical and Nursing Dictionary, 1983:483.

21. Dokheel, TM. "An epidemic of childhood diabetes in the United States." *Diabetes Care* 1993;16:1601-1611.

22. Gardner, S., et al. "Rising incidence of insulin dependent diabetes in children under 5 years in Oxford region: time trend analysis." *British Medical Journal* 1997;315:713-716.

23. Classen, JB., et al. "Association between type 1 diabetes and Hib vaccine." *British Medical Journal* 1999;319:1133.

24. Classen, JB., et al. "Clustering of Cases of Insulin Dependent Diabetes (IDDM) Occurring Three Years After Haemophilus Influenza B (HiB) Immunization Support Causal Relationship Between Immunization and IDDM." *Autoimmunity* 2002;35(4):247-53.

25. Vaccine Safety Website. "Haemophilus vaccine study in Finland supports a relationship between vaccines and diabetes." www.vaccines.net/newpage16.htm (Last accessed: August 12, 2009).

26. See Notes 23-25.

27. PRNewswire. "Haemophilus meningitis vaccine linked to diabetes increase; many diabetics may be eligible for compensation" (May 7, 1999). www.islet.org/forum011/messages/7958.htm (Last accessed: August 12, 2009).

28. Ibid.

29. Ibid.

30. Classen, JB. "Public should be told that vaccines may have long term adverse effects." *British Medical Journal* 1999;318:193.

31. See Note 23.

32. Thinktwice Global Vaccine Institute. Unsolicited case report submitted by a concerned parent. www.thinktwice.com

33. See Note 15.

34. CDC. "Current trends FDA workshop on Haemophilus b polysaccharide vaccine..." *MMWR* (August 21, 1987);36(32):529-31.

35. See Notes 3, 4 and 9.

36. Weiss, R. "Meningitis Vaccine Stirs Controversy," *Sci News* (Oct 24, 1987);132:260.

37. American Academy of Pediatrics. "Policy Statement: Haemophilus b poly-saccharide vaccine (HbPV)," *AAP News* (November 1987):7.

38. Black, S., et al. "Efficacy of Haemophilus influenzae type b capsular polysaccharide vaccine," *Pediatric Infectious Disease Journal* 1988;7:149-156.

39. Harrison, LH., et al. "A day care-based study of the efficacy of Haemophilus influenzae type b polysaccharide vaccine." *J of the American Med Assoc* 1988;260:1413-1418.

40. Osterholm, MT., et al. "Lack of efficacy of Haemophilus b polysaccharide vaccine in Minnesota." *J of the American Medical Association* 1988;260:1423-1428.

41. Shapiro, ED., et al. "The protective efficacy of Haemophilus influenzae polysaccharide vaccine." *J of the American Medical Assoc.* 1988;260:1419-1422.

42. Hiner, EE., et al. "Spectrum of disease due to Haemophilus influenzae type b occurring in vaccinated children." *J of Infectious Disease* 1988;158(2):343-48.

43. Daum, RS. et al. "Decline in serum antibody to the capsule of Haemophilus influenzae type b in the immediate postimmunization period." *J of Pediatrics* 1989;1114:742-47.

44. Marchant, DD., et al. "Depression of anticapsular antibody after immunization with Haemophilus influenzae type b polysaccharide-diphtheria conjugate vaccine." *Pediatric Infectious Disease Journal* 1989;320:75-81.

45. Sood, SK., et al. "Disease caused by Haemophilus influenzae type b in the immediate period after homologous immunization: immunologic investigation." *Pediatrics* 1990;85 (4 Pt 2):698-704.

46. See Note 19.

47. Zwillich, Todd. "Hib rates in U.S. children higher among minorities than whites." *Reuters Medical News* (August 18, 2000).

Pneumococcal

What is pneumococcal disease?
Pneumococcal disease, or *streptococcus pneumoniae,* is a serious bacterial illness that can cause meningitis, pneumonia, ear infections, sinusitis, and bacteremia (an infection of the blood). The pneumococcal pathogen consists of approximately 90 different strains.

How prevalent and serious is pneumococcal disease?
During the 1980s and 1990s, the annual incidence of pneumococcal disease in the United States was an estimated 10 to 30 cases per 100,000 persons. In children under 5 years old, about 15 percent of cases are meningitis while the rest are usually blood infections. According to the CDC, this translated into about 700 cases of meningitis, 13,000 blood infections, and approximately 200 deaths annually.

Who is most susceptible to pneumococcal disease?
Persons 65 years and older, children under two years of age, immuno-compromised adults, and the chronically ill are at greatest risk of contracting pneumococcal disease. Most healthy children are not at risk. In fact, according to the Red Book Report of the Committee on Infectious Diseases published by the American Academy of Pediatrics, "[Pneumococcal infections in children] are more likely to occur when predisposing conditions exist, including immunoglobulin deficiency, Hodgkin's disease, congenital or acquired immunodeficiency (including HIV), nephrotic syndrome, some viral upper respiratory tract infections, splenic dysfunction, splenectomy and organ transplantation."[1]

The pneumococcal vaccine:
In February 2010, the FDA approved a new diphtheria-conjugated pneumococcal vaccine—Prevnar 13—for children 6 weeks through 5 years of age. Prevnar 13 is made to protect against 13 of the approximately 90 different pneumococcal strains capable of causing bacterial disease. This vaccine will replace Prevnar (PCV7), introduced ten years earlier.
- Prevnar 13—A solution of 13 *Streptococcus pneumoniae* serotypes "grown in a soy peptone broth." Each dose contains 125mcg of aluminum and polysorbate 80. Produced by Wyeth. Given in 4 doses.[2]
- Prevnar (PCV7)—Manufactured with 7 pneumococcal strains and 125mcg of aluminum.[3]

Safety

Studies documenting systemic reactions to the pneumococcal vaccine confirm that many children experience diarrhea, vomiting, irritability, a rash or hives, and tenderness at the injection site "interfering with limb movement."[4-6] In fact, according to the American Academy of Pediatrics...

> *"Available data suggest that [the pneumococcal vaccine] may prove to be among the most reactogenic vaccine of those currently used."[7]*
> —**American Academy of Pediatrics**

Data sheets produced by the vaccine manufacturer list several serious adverse reactions that occurred during pre-licensure trials of the vaccine. Although the manufacturer does not admit a causative relationship between the vaccine and many of these reactions, parents who are considering this shot for their children may wish to weigh the implications. Such reactions included 162 visits to the emergency room and 24 hospitalizations within 3 days of a dose for various ailments, such as congestive heart failure, aplastic anemia, autoimmune disease, diabetes mellitus, neutropenia, thrombocytopenia, pneumonia, bronchiolitis, colitis, otitis media, asthma, wheezing, croup, seizures, hypotonic-hyporesponsive episode, and several deaths, many of which were attributed to SIDS. In fact, the vaccine manufacturer admits that "there have been spontaneous reports of apnea (temporary cessation of breathing) in temporal association" with the administration of this shot.[8] Additional adverse reactions identified after this vaccine was marketed include seizures, blood and lymphatic system disorders (lymphadenopathy), immune system disorders, such as broncho-spasms, and anaphylactic reactions, including face edema and shock.[9]

The pneumococcal vaccine and DIABETES:

Dr. Barthelow Classen, an immunologist at Classen Immunotherapies, testified before the FDA that the pneumococcal vaccine "could cause a major epidemic of diabetes."[10] He presented data in the *British Medical Journal* and *Autoimmunity* showing a statistical link between the Hib shot and diabetes.[11,12] He claims the pneumococcal vaccine is technologically similar to the Hib vaccine, and calculates that it will cause 28,000 cases of diabetes every year in the USA alone. "These cases of diabetes may not occur until 3½ to 10 years following the shot."[13,14] Classen also declared that the risks greatly exceed the benefits, and told the FDA that it should not license this vaccine until it can be given without inducing diabetes.[15]

Pneumococcal Vaccine—VAERS Case Reports

The case reports below were taken directly from the FDA's Vaccine Adverse Event Reporting System (VAERS).[16] They are just a small sample of the potential harm associated with the pneumococcal vaccine.

▸244320: A 4-month-old girl received the pneumococcal vaccine, developed pneumococcal infection (*streptococcus pneumoniae*), and died.

▸169943: A 4-month-old boy received Prevnar, went into a coma and died the following day.

▸216583: A 4-month-old girl received Prevnar and died the following day. The autopsy report listed SIDS.

▸232422: A 4-month-old girl received Prevnar and was hospitalized the next day with "hypothermia, hypotension, and acidosis." She died 2 days later.

▸273844: An 8-month-old girl received Prevnar at 10 in the morning and was found dead in her room at 3 in the afternoon.

▸227847: A 9-month-old boy received Prevnar, developed "breathlessness" and died 6 days later due to "congestive cardiomyopathy."

▸240197: A 9-month-old girl received Prevnar and experienced apnea, cyanosis and cardiac arrest 3 days later.

▸158751: A 10-month-old boy received Prevnar and died of "cardi-pulmonary arrest" the following day.

▸231321: Four days after receiving Prevnar, a 10-month-old female developed abdominal distention, apnea, hypoxia, bronchitis and respiratory failure. She died in the emergency room.

▸217931: A 15-month-old girl received the pneumococcal vaccine (Prevnar) "and subsequently developed hemolytic-uremic syndrome and pneumococcal pneumonia." Day 3 of hospitalization brought sudden death.

▸270765: A 17-month-old girl received the pneumococcal vaccine. Two days later, she developed pneumococcal meningitis and died the following day.

▸271911: A 20-month-old boy received the pneumococcal vaccine and subsequently experienced "pneumococcal meningitis, drug ineffective, cardio-respiratory failure, and septic shock."

▸247661: A 1-year-old girl received the pneumococcal vaccine (Prevnar) and subsequently "experienced pneumococcal meningitis, pneumococcal bacteremia, pneumococcal sepsis, drug ineffective, and cerebral infarction." She remained in intensive care for 17 days until she died.

▸244321: A 1½-year-old girl developed pneumococcal bacteremia and died after receiving the pneumococcal vaccine.

226284: A 3-year-old boy received the pneumococcal vaccine, subsequently developed pneumococcal meningitis, and died.

▸238155: A 3-year-old child received Prevnar and died 2 days later from "cardiac respiratory shutdown."

Case Reports by Parents

Many parents believe the pneumococcal vaccine caused adverse reactions in their children.[17] Here are three of their stories:

▸ *"I had a baby that was perfectly healthy, happy, okay until she got her Prevnar vaccine. Thirty hours later, she's in the hospital having seizures that they can't stop. You're not going to tell me it's not related to the vaccine."* [This child slipped in an out of a coma for 45 days—with tremors that shook her little body most of the time—until she died.]

▸ *"My daughter was given Prevnar at 9 months. Three days later she threw her head back, her eyes rolled back in her head, and she was unresponsive. She continued to do this for the next two years. We were also told she had cerebral palsy, although she had no symptoms of any health problems until she received the shots. She was normal until this happened. She was even rolling over at two months and crawling at six months. She was starting to talk at seven months. She quit talking and quit walking altogether. Thank you for listening. My daughter will not receive any more vaccinations ever!"*

▸ *"I am a mother of 18-month-old twins. Both received the Prevnar shot and have been experiencing daily reactions: wheezing, fever, rash, and diarrhea. My son was taken to the emergency room by ambulance within 12 hours of injection for a seizure. He was taken a second time the following morning. Neither child could walk the first 48 hours after the shot. They reverted to crawling. My son was in the midst of his 3rd seizure, this one lasting much longer and more severe than the first ones. We rushed him to the ER where he underwent a CAT Scan and Spinal Tap. He was transported to another hospital where he could be evaluated by a specialist, and underwent EEG. According to the doctors, there are no hidden ailments causing these seizures; the suspected culprit is the Prevnar injection."*

Efficacy

Vaccine efficacy was determined by calculating the percentage of vaccinated children achieving a pre-determined immune response—as measured by antibody levels—to the 13 individual pneumococcal strains included in the vaccine. On this basis, efficacy ranged from 64 percent (strain 3) to 98 percent (strains 7F, 14, 19A, and 19F). However...

"Prevnar 13 will not protect against streptococcus pneumoniae serotypes that are not in the vaccine or serotypes unrelated to those in the vaccine."[18]
—The vaccine manufacturer

How does STRAIN REPLACEMENT influence efficacy?

The pneumococcal vaccine is not only ineffective against more than 75 different pneumococcal strains (the ones not included in the vaccine), they may also be gaining strength. Scientists have known for some time that *streptococcus pneumoniae* are subject to changes by "recombination." This has caused researchers to issue warnings that pneumococcal vaccines only targeting some strains of the disease "may increase carriage of and disease from serotypes not included in the vaccine."[19,20] Scientists writing for the *Journal of Molecular Microbiology* concur, and conclude that "this has implications for the long-term efficacy of conjugate pneumococcal vaccines that will protect against only a limited number of serotypes."[21]

In 2007, the *Pediatric Infectious Disease Journal* published data confirming "serotype replacement," where less prevalent (but more severe) pneumococcal strains replace the limited number of strains that are targeted by the vaccine.[22] During 2000, the year in which Prevnar was licensed, 65 percent of all pneumoccocal cases were caused by strains included in the vaccine. By 2004, just 27 percent of all pneumococcal cases were caused by vaccine strains; *73 percent of all cases were now due to non-vaccine strains!*[23] Furthermore, these non-vaccine strains are more resistant to antibiotics and multi-drug treatments. In addition, *vaccine* strains of pneumococcal disease have become more resistant to antibiotics as well.[24]

In 2007, the *Journal of the American Medical Association* also published data showing that non-vaccine strains of pneumococcal disease are replacing the strains targeted by the vaccine. For example, ever since Prevnar was introduced, "the incidence of non-PCV7 serotype disease more than doubled among Alaska Native children."[25] In addition, the new strains are more dangerous. Compared with illness prior to Prevnar vaccination, "current cases are more likely to be hospitalized and to be diagnosed with pneumonia and empyema"[26] (a life-threatening infection causing pus and fluid to accumulate in the lung cavity).

The pneumococcal vaccine and EAR INFECTIONS:

The vaccine industry promotes this shot as being protective against middle ear infections (acute otitis media). However, the pneumococcal vaccine is only indicated for vaccination against otitis media "caused by serotypes included in the vaccine." The manufacturer admits that "children who received Prevnar appear to be at *increased* risk of otitis media due to pneumococcal serotypes not represented in the vaccine." In fact, the vaccine has *no statistical efficacy* when measured against *all* acute otitis media episodes.[27]

Notes

1. Red Book report of the Committee on Infectious Diseases, 23rd edition. *American Academy of Pediatrics* 1994:371.

2. Wyeth. "Prevnar 13 (Pneumococcal 13-valent Conjugate Vaccine [Diphtheria CRM197 Protein])." February 2010.

3. Wyeth. "Prevnar (Pneumococcal 7-valent Conjugate Vaccine)." October 2008.

4. See Notes 2 and 3.

5. Black, S., et al. "Efficacy, safety and immunogenicity of heptavalent pneumococcal conjugate vaccine in children." Northern California Kaiser Permanente Vaccine Study Center Group. *Pediatric Infectious Disease J* (March 2000);19(3):187-95.

6. Black, S., et al. "Efficacy of heptavalent conjugate pneumococcal vaccine (Lederle Laboratories) in 37,000 infants and children." Results of the Northern California Kaiser Permanente Efficacy Trial. 36th ICAAC, San Diego, CA. (September 24-27, 1998).

7. Overturf, G. "Technical report: prevention of pneumococcal infections, including the use of pneumococcal conjugate and polysaccharide vaccines and antibiotic prophylaxis (RE9960)." *American Academy of Pediatrics and the Committee on Infectious Diseases.*

8. See Notes 2 and 3.

9. Ibid.

10. Press release. "FDA told pneumococcal vaccine likely to cause epidemic of diabetes." (Nov. 8, 1999).

11. Classen, JB., et al. "Association between type 1 diabetes and Hib vaccine." *British Medical Journal* 1999;319:1133.

12. Classen, JB., et al. "Clustering of Cases of Insulin Dependent Diabetes (IDDM) Occurring Three Years After Haemophilus Influenza B (HiB) Immunization Support Causal Relationship Between Immunization and IDDM." *Autoimmunity* 2002;35(4):247-53.

13. Classen, B. "New 'Tuskegee-like experiment' planned with pneumococcal vaccine." www.vaccines.net/pneumoco.htm

14. See Note 10.

15. Ibid.

16. U.S. Department of Health and Human Services. "Vaccine Adverse Event Reporting System (VAERS)." www.hhs.gov

17. Thinktwice Global Vaccine Institute. Unsolicited case reports submitted by concerned parents. www.thinktwice.com

18. See Note 2.

19. Lipsitch, M. "Bacterial vaccines and serotype replacement: lessons from haemophilus influenzae and prospects for streptococcus pneumoniae." *Emerging Infectious Diseases* (May-Jun 1999);5(3):336-45.

20. Lipsitch, M. "Vaccination against colonizing bacteria with multiple serotypes." *Proceedings of the National Academy of Sciences* (June 1997);94(12):6571-76.

21. Coffey, TJ., et al. "Recombinational exchanges at the capsular polysaccharide biosynthetic locus lead to frequent serotype changes among natural isolates of Streptococcus pneumoniae." *Journal of Molecular Microbiology* (January 1998); 27(1):73-83.

22. Farrell, DJ., et al. "Increased antimicrobial resistance among nonvaccine serotypes of *streptococcus pneumoniae* in the pediatric population after the introduction of 7-valent pneumococcal vaccine in the United States." *Pediatric Infectious Disease Journal* 2007; 26(2):123-28.

23. Ibid.

24. Ibid.

25. Singleton, RJ., et al. "Invasive pneumococcal disease caused by nonvaccine serotypes among Alaska native children with high levels of 7-valent pneumococcal conjugate vaccine coverage." *JAMA* (April 25, 2007);297:1784-92.

26. Ibid.

27. See Notes 2 and 3.

Meningococcus

What is meningococcal disease?

Meningococcal disease, or *neisseria meningitidis,* is a serious bacterial illness that can cause meningitis and meningococcemia, or septicaemia (blood poisoning). High fever, headache and stiff neck are common symptoms of meningitis in anyone over the age of two years. In babies, the classic symptoms may be more difficult to notice. The meningococcal pathogen consists of at least 13 different strains.

How prevalent and serious is meningococcal disease?

Meningococcal disease is relatively rare. According to the CDC, 1400 to 2800 cases occur each year in the United States, a rate of approximately 1 or 2 cases for every 200,000 people.[1] Of 14 million students in colleges nationwide, about 100 get this disease each year.[2] About 10 percent of the population carries the bacteria in its nonpathogenic form. None of the bacteria that cause meningitis—including *neisseria meningitidis*—are as contagious as ailments like the common cold or flu. Bacterial meningitis can be treated with antibiotics. The case fatality rate is about 10 percent. About 15 percent of cases result in hearing loss or other sequelae.

Who is most susceptible to meningococcal disease?

People with weak immune systems or suffering from a chronic underlying medical condition, are most susceptible to meningococcal disease. Infants and children have disproportionately higher rates of this disease, but nearly two-thirds of all cases occur in persons aged 15 years and older.[3] Anyone having direct contact with an infected person's oral secretions (such as a boyfriend or girlfriend) may be at increased risk of acquiring the infection. College students living on-campus, especially freshmen, appear to be at higher risk than those residing off campus. However, incidence among college students "usually is similar to or somewhat lower than that observed among persons in the general population of similar age."[4]

The meningococcal vaccine:

In January 2005, a new vaccine for meningococcal disease—Menactra (or MCV4)—was licensed by the FDA. It is designed to protect against 4 of the 13 distinct strains of meningococcus. The CDC recommends this shot for all adolescents 11 to 18 years of age.

- Menactra—Contains *Neisseria meningitidis* strains A, C, Y and W-135 antigens "individually conjugated to diphtheria toxoid protein." Each dose also contains sodium chloride, sodium phosphate and formaldehyde. Produced by Sanofi Pasteur.[5]

Safety

In the United Kingdom, a nationwide meningococcal vaccine campaign was initiated in November 1999. Less than one year later, by September 2000, the British Committee on Safety of Medicines had already received more than 7,500 Yellow Card reports—suspected adverse reactions—after the meningococcal shot, including at least 12 deaths. The British government tried convincing the public that most of the deaths were caused by sudden infant death syndrome (SIDS).[6] In one study of Menactra among persons 11-18 years of age, approximately half of the participants experienced at least one systemic adverse reaction, and nearly 5 percent (about one of every 20 people vaccinated) experienced at least one *severe* systemic reaction. Non-systemic reactions were common as well.[7]

According to the vaccine manufacturer, several neurological and immunological disorders have been reported in vaccine recipients after Menactra was brought to market: Guillain-Barré syndrome, facial palsy, transverse myelitis, encephalomyelitis, anaphylactic reactions, wheezing, difficulty breathing, urticaria and hypotension.[8]

MCV4 and GUILLAIN-BARRÉ SYNDROME:

Shortly after this new vaccine (Menactra, or MCV4) was officially certified as safe by the FDA and placed on the market for mass consumption, several people were stricken with Guillain-Barré syndrome (GBS) following their shots.[9] GBS is a serious neurologic disorder involving inflammatory demyelination of nerves. Symptoms begin with tingling sensations in the legs, arms, and upper body. As the disease progresses, the muscles weaken or can no longer be used, there is a loss of mobility, and in severe cases, the individual may be paralyzed. Sensory abnormalities and paralysis of respiratory muscles can also occur. About 20 percent of hospitalized patients can have prolonged disability and a smaller percentage of patients will die from GBS.[10]

The case reports on the following page occurred in the Eastern United States within a six-week period. All of the victims were 17 or 18 years old. The onset of symptoms was 14 to 31 days after Menactra vaccination.[11]

MCV4 and Guillain-Barré Syndrome

▶Case 1: A male aged 18 years was vaccinated with MCV4; 15 days later, he experienced tingling in his feet and hands.... Sixteen days after vaccination, he was hospitalized.... He was observed for 3 days, discharged, and then readmitted 2 days later with bilateral facial weakness and increasing lower extremity weakness. Patellar, triceps, and biceps deep tendon reflexes were absent. Nerve conduction studies...revealed worsening motor nerve conduction velocities consistent with Guillain-Barré syndrome.

▶Case 2: A male aged 17 years was vaccinated with MCV4; approximately 25 days later, he had difficulty walking, followed by difficulty moving from a standing to a seated position.... Thirty-two days after vaccination, he was hospitalized with bilateral muscle weakness of upper and lower extremities with absent deep tendon reflexes.

▶Case 3: A female aged 17 years.... Fourteen days after vaccination with MCV4, she reported numbness of toes and tongue, and had a lump in her throat. These symptoms were followed by numbness of thighs and fingertips, arm weakness, inability to run, difficulty walking, and falling. Sixteen days after vaccination, she was hospitalized, and neurologic examination revealed decreased tone, weakness of both arms and legs, and reflexes reduced or absent in ankles, knees and arms.

▶Case 4: A female aged 18 years was vaccinated with MCV4.... Thirty-one days after vaccination, the patient reported numbness of legs and had trouble standing on her toes. The next morning she could not stand. The patient was admitted to the hospital and physical examination revealed decreased muscle strength in ankles and wrists bilaterally, and reduced biceps, knee, and ankle deep tendon reflexes.

▶Case 5: A female aged 18 years was vaccinated with MCV4; 14 days later, she experienced heaviness in her legs when walking upstairs. During the next 8 days, her difficulty walking around continued, and she had bilateral leg pain. Subsequently, she reported headache, back and neck pain, vomiting, and tingling in both hands. She became unable to walk and...was hospitalized for progressive weakness and inability to walk.... Weakness progressed to include paralysis of arms, difficulty swallowing, and respiratory compromise.

On October 20, 2006, the FDA and CDC alerted consumers and healthcare providers about 17 confirmed cases of GBS following routine administration of the Menactra vaccine. These cases were in older teens and people 20 years of age or greater. GBS occurred within six weeks following injection with Menactra.[12] At least two law firms started representing victims of the shot.[13,14] Nevertheless, this vaccine was not removed from the market. Instead, the vaccine manufacturer updated the package insert "to reflect that GBS has been reported in association with the vaccine."[15] The general populace was also informed that the FDA and CDC "are continuing to monitor the situation."[16] However, just two weeks later, the CDC Advisory Committee on Immunization Practices (ACIP) recommended "resumption of immunization for all groups previously recommended to receive routine Menactra immunization."[17]

Efficacy

Menactra vaccine efficacy was determined by providing the shot to a small group of people and then measuring the number of meningococcal-fighting antibodies—to strains A, C, Y and W-135—produced in the blood. If this number meets or exceeds a pre-established "protective level" then the vaccine is considered effective. By this criterion, Menactra is considered "non-inferior" to Menomune, an earlier meningococcal vaccine. However, "measurable levels of antibodies against the group A and C...decrease markedly during the first 3 years following a single dose of vaccine."[18,19]

Authorities often promote the meningococcal vaccine by publicizing the annual number of cases and deaths caused by the disease. However, this is deceitful because the vaccine will not prevent many of these unfortunate tragedies. This is because the meningococcal vaccine is only indicated for the prevention of meningococcal disease caused by 4 of the 13 known strains: A, C, Y and W-135. The meningococcal vaccine does not contain—and will not protect against—the B strain of meningococcus, the most prevalent cause of meningococcal disease in developed countries. For example, the King County, Washington Health Department reported that from January 2000 through 2006, 64 percent of all strain-identified cases of meningococcal disease among teenagers could not have been prevented with a meningococcal vaccine because they were caused by a serotype not included in the shot.[20]

The B strain is also the most virulent of all the strains, the most common serotype causing meningococcal meningitis and a disproportionate number of fatalities.[21] For example, during the 2002/2003 epidemiological year, 82 percent of all laboratory confirmed cases of meningococcal disease—and 73 percent of all meningococcal deaths—in the United Kingdom, Wales and Northern Ireland, were caused by strain B.[22] In France, 58 percent of all meningococcal cases between 1999 and 2002 were from serotype B.[23] In the U.S., approximately one-third of all meningococcal cases, and more than 50 percent of all cases in infants, are caused by the B strain.[24,25]

The meningococcal vaccine and VIRULENT STRAINS:

The meningococcal vaccine may be causing other strains of the disease to become more dangerous. For example, in a recent issue of the *Journal of Clinical Microbiology,* vaccine researchers believe that a cluster of fierce, new "hypervirulent" B strain meningococcal cases "is possibly related to the mass immunization campaign" conducted earlier in the region.[26] Recent research in the *Indian Journal of Medical Microbiology* affirmed that "meningococci have the capacity to exchange the genetic material responsible for capsule production and thereby switch from serogroup B to C or vice versa." In fact, the study authors conclude that "capsule switching may become an important mechanism of virulence with the widespread use of vaccines that provide serogroup-specific protection."[27] In other words, vaccines that only protect against certain strains—Menactra only protects against strains A, C, Y and W-135—could allow other non-vaccine strains to gain in both frequency and strength. A recent study in *Clinical Infectious Diseases* found that "the prevalence of meningococci with reduced susceptibility to penicillin is increasing."[28]

Vaccine Failures: Prospective recipients of the meningococcal vaccine should know that it will not protect against bacterial meningitis caused by pneumococcus, Hib, or newly emerging strains. Thus, when a person is vaccinated and still contracts bacterial disease, it will be difficult to determine whether the vaccine failed—or if the disease was actually *caused* by the vaccine, by a strain not included in the shot, or by a completely different bacterial pathogen. The following story typifies the possibilities:

"Following my meningitis shot, I ended up in the hospital with a major infection that attacked every area of my system. Doctors did a lumbar puncture on me. This involved freezing my mid-section so they could insert a large needle into the pit of my spinal cord. Their diagnosis was meningitis. I remained hospitalized for 3 weeks. They wouldn't even consider that my meningitis shot could have caused my nearly fatal disease."[29]
—**Recipient of the meningococcal vaccine**

Is the meningococcal vaccine mandatory?

The American Academy of Pediatrics (AAP) recently declared that "universal vaccination [with meningococcal vaccine] is not necessary."[30] The CDC conducted a financial analysis of vaccination for all college students and determined that it is not likely to be cost-effective. For example, vaccination of college freshmen who live in dormitories might prevent "16 to 30 cases of meningococcal disease" each year at an estimated cost of more than $600,000 per case![31] Instead, a national campaign is being aimed at middle school students, a larger, more cost-effective cohort. Of course, if this vaccine is mandatory in your state for school entry, or is required for enrollment in a specific college, exemptions are possible.

Notes

1. CDC. "Prevention and control of meningococcal disease." *MMWR* (May 27, 2005):1-21.

2. CDC. "Meningococcal disease and college students." *MMWR* (Jun 30, 2000):11-20.

3. Raghunathan, PL., et al. "Opportunities for control of meningococcal disease in the US." *Annual Review of Medicine, CDC.* (February 2004); Vol. 55:333-353.

4. See Note 1.

5. Sanofi Pasteur. "Menactra (Groups A, C, Y, W-135) Polysaccharide Diphtheria Toxoid Conjugate Vaccine." April 2008.

6. Woodman, R. "Meningitis C vaccine not responsible for deaths." *Reuters Medical News* (Sept 5, 2000).

7. See Note 1.

8. See Note 5.

9. CDC. "Guillain-Barré syndrome among recipients of Menactra meningococcal conjugate vaccine: US, June-July 2005." *MMWR* (Oct. 6, 2005);54(Dispatch):1-3.

10. See Notes 5 and 9.

11. See Note 9.

12. FDA. "FDA and CDC update information on Menactra meningococcal vaccine and Guillain Barré syndrome." www.fda.gov (October 20, 2006).

13. Farrin, JS. "Rare disorder reported with Menactra drug recall alerts." James Scott Farrin, NC Personal Injury Lawyers. www.farrin.com (October 20, 2006).

14. See Note 12.

15. See Note 9.

16. See Note 12.

17. King County Public Health. "Immunization program: meningococcal conjugate (Menactra) vaccine supply update." www.metrokc.gov (Updated: Dec 4, 2006).

18. Sanofi Pasteur. "Menomune (Meningococcal Polysaccharide Vaccine, Groups A, C, Y and W-135 Combined)." December 2005.

19. See Notes 1 and 5.

20. See Note 17.

21. Hincapie, M., et al. "Neisseria Meningitidis." *Brown University.* www.brown.edu

22. British Health Protection Agency. "Enhanced surveillance of meningococcal disease: national annual report, July 2002—June 2003." www.hpa.org.uk

23. Antignac, A., et al. "Neisseria meningitidis strains isolated from invasive infections... phenotypes and antibiotic susceptibility patterns." *Clin Infec Dis* 2003;37:912+.

24. See Note 1.

25. National Institutes of Health. "Safety and immunogenicity study of group B meningococcal vaccine..." *Walter Reed Army Inst of Research.* clinicaltrials.gov

26. Law, D., et al. "Invasive meningococcal disease in Québec, Canada, due to an emerging clone of ST-269 serogroup B meningococci..." *J Clin Microbio* (Aug 2006);44(8):2743-49.

27. Manchanda, V., et al. "Meningococcal disease: history, epidemiology, pathogenesis, clinical manifestations, diagnosis..." *Indian J of Med Microbiology* 2006;24, Issue 1:7-19.

28. See Note 23.

29. Thinktwice Global Vaccine Institute. Unsolicited case report. www.thinktwice.com

30. CDC. "Meningococcal disease and college students." *MMWR* (June 30, 2000); 49(RR07):11-20.

31. See Note 1.

Rotavirus

What is rotavirus?

Rotavirus is a common cause of diarrhea and vomiting in children. It occurs most often in the winter months. Symptoms typically last from 3 to 8 days and may include a fever and abdominal pain. Although babies 6 months to 2 years are most vulnerable to rotavirus infection, nearly all children are exposed to this contagious microbe at least once by the time they are 5 years old. The illness causes partial immunity because repeat infections are less severe. In most cases, rotavirus is mild enough that parents can care for their children at home. However, in severe cases dehydration and death are possible. Over 80 percent of all rotavirus deaths occur in poor countries where babies are malnourished and there is limited access to advanced healthcare. In the United States, about 20 deaths per year are attributed to this disease.

Treatment mainly consists of preventing dehydration by giving fluids until the disease runs its course. In serious cases, frequent vomiting makes oral hydration ineffective. Babies unable to keep down liquids risk dying from dehydration and require intravenous fluids.

The rotavirus vaccine:

- RotaTeq—A live-virus, oral vaccine for infants under 32 weeks of age. Designed to protect against four of the most common strains of rotavirus. Each dose contains "live reassortant rotaviruses...isolated from human and bovine hosts...propagated in Vero cells" (from the kidneys of African green monkeys). Each dose also contains sucrose, sodium citrate, sodium phosphate monobasic monohydrate, sodium hydroxide, polysorbate 80, cell culture media, "and trace amounts of fetal bovine serum." Produced by Merck. U.S. licensed in 2006. Given in 3 doses.[1]
- Rotarix— A live-virus, oral vaccine for infants under 24 weeks of age. Designed to protect against four strains of rotavirus. Derived from "the human 89-12 strain...propagated on Vero cells." Each dose also contains sodium chloride, sodium phosphate, sodium pyruvate, sodium hydrogenocarbonate, calcium carbonate, calcium chloride, potassium chloride, ferric (III) nitrate, magnesium sulfate, phenol red, L-glutamine, sorbitol, sucrose and xanthan. Developed by GSK. U.S. licensed in 2008. Given in 2 doses.[2]

Safety

Can the rotavirus vaccine cause SEVERE INTESTINAL DAMAGE?
The RotaTeq manufacturer warns parents to remain alert to the possibility of intussusception—severe intestinal damage—in their babies following use of this vaccine:

> *"If your child develops sudden abdominal pain, vomiting, blood in their stools or other changes in their bowel movements, it may be a sign of a serious problem. You should call the doctor immediately."*[3]
> —The Vaccine Manufacturer

A study of this vaccine was recently published in the *New England Journal of Medicine*. Within this study, a safety substudy was conducted to look for "potential cases of intussusception" that were initially denied by investigators. Babies who received the RotaTeq vaccine had a greater than threefold risk of hematochezia when compared to babies who received the placebo.[4] Hematochezia is the passage of bloody stools from the rectum, associated with lower gastrointestinal bleeding.

The case reports on the following page—of intussusception and/or hematochezia after receiving the RotaTeq vaccine—were taken directly from the FDA's Vaccine Adverse Event Reporting System (VAERS).[5] They are just a small sample of the potential harm associated with this vaccine. (Case numbers precede report summaries.)

Is the RotaTeq vaccine causing SEIZURES?
In placebo-controlled clinical trials of the RotaTeq vaccine, "seizures" and "seizures reported as serious adverse experiences" occurred at higher rates in vaccine recipients. Twice as many babies who received RotaTeq (as compared to babies who received placebo) had seizures within 7 days after any dose. Seizures reported as serious adverse experiences occurred at a rate of 510 out of one million in the placebo group versus 750 out of one million in the vaccine group.[6] Thus, thousands of babies every year will be stricken with serious seizures that could have been avoided by declining this vaccine.

Additional RotaTeq vaccine safety issues:
More than 71,000 infants were evaluated in three placebo-controlled clinical trials that were ultimately used to license RotaTeq. Here is a summary of adverse reactions that occurred at a statistically higher rate

RotaTeq Vaccine: VAERS Case Reports of Intussusception

►266155: An 11-week-old female was vaccinated with RotaTeq and developed severe vomiting. The infant vomited so much that she was hospitalized. An ultrasound diagnosis of intussusception was made.

►266161: A 2-month-old baby received the RotaTeq vaccine and 6 days later was diagnosed with intussusception requiring surgical reduction.

►279032: A 3-month-old started vomiting, and had bloody stools, after receiving RotaTeq. The infant was transferred from one hospital to another with symptoms of hematochezia, intussusception, and intestinal obstruction.

►268405: A 4-month-old baby developed intestinal obstruction 2 days after receiving the RotaTeq vaccine. Abdomen surgery revealed "intussusception with gangrenous ascending and transverse colon."

►269344: A 4-month-old received the RotaTeq vaccine and subsequently developed intussusception and gastrointestinal necrosis. The infant required "surgery for resection at necrotic bowel."

among babies who received the RotaTeq vaccine when compared to babies who received a placebo.[7] This list includes adverse events that occurred within 6 weeks of any dose:

- **Diarrhea.** This is the most common symptom of rotavirus, the main reason to seek protection against this disease. However, in the studies used as a basis for licensing this vaccine, diarrhea occurred statistically more often in recipients of the vaccine than in babies who never received a single dose.
- **Vomiting.** Again, statistically more common in vaccine recipients.
- **Otitis media.** This is a painful inflammation or infection of the middle ear. Untreated otitis media may lead to permanent hearing impairment.
- **Bronchospasm.** An abnormal constriction of the respiratory airway causing difficult and labored breathing. This condition is a chief feature of asthma and bronchitis. A cough and wheezing are common.
- **Nasopharyngitis.** This is a viral infectious disease of the upper respiratory system, often accompanied by a sore throat and runny nose.
- **Dermatitis.** The *New England Journal of Medicine* safety substudy found that dermatitis occurred more often among vaccine recipients than among the group receiving placebo. Dermatitis, called eczema as well, is an inflammation of the skin. It is caused by an allergic reaction to allergens.

Serious adverse reactions linked to the Rotarix vaccine:
Clinical studies have found statistical correlations between the Rotarix vaccine and higher rates of **death** (pneumonia-related), **convulsions** (epilepsy, grand mal, status epilepticus, and tonic), **bronchitis,** and **Kawasaki disease** (which often leads to heart disease and sudden death)[8-15] In addition, more parents of babies who received the vaccine (versus parents of babies in the placebo group) discontinued the study due to serious adverse events.[16]

Is the Rotarix vaccine causing an increased rate of BABY DEATHS?

In the clinical studies used to evaluate the safety of the Rotarix vaccine, *vaccinated babies died at a much higher rate than non-vaccinated babies* —mainly due to a statistically significant increase in pneumonia-related fatalities: a death rate of 18.5 versus 14.5 per 10,000.[17] In other words, for every one million babies who receive this vaccine, we can expect 1,850 to die. However, if we leave them unvaccinated, just 1,450 will die—400 babies per every million would be saved by *not* vaccinating them! In addition, twice as many vaccinated babies died from *diarrhea* when compared to the non-vaccinated babies.[18]

Efficacy

The RotaTeq vaccine is designed to protect against four strains of rotavirus: serotypes G1-G4. Researchers would consider the vaccine a success if it could be proven "efficacious in preventing wild-type G1-G4 rotavirus gastroenteritis occurring 14 or more days after completion of the three-dose series through the first full rotavirus season after vaccination."[19] Using this definition, the vaccine was rated 74 percent effective "against any grade of severity" of rotavirus, and 98 percent effective against "severe" cases of the ailment.[20] (These figures are 87 percent and 96 percent, respectively, for Rotarix.)[21] In addition, the vaccine reduced hospitalizations "for rotavirus gastroenteritis caused by serotypes G1, G2, G3, and G4"—the strains included in the vaccine.[22]

Does the rotavirus vaccine protect against all types of diarrhea?

No. Parents should realize that rotavirus vaccines will not protect against diarrhea caused by rotavirus strains not included in the vaccine. The vaccine is designed to protect against four strains of rotavirus, but several rotavirus strains have been identified. Diarrhea can also be caused by other distinct pathogens. For example, astrovirus infection occurs worldwide and is a significant cause of diarrhea. One study conducted in England showed that astroviruses were the most frequent viral cause of infectious intestinal disease.[23] Calicivirus infection is associated with diarrhea and vomiting lasting several days. Caliciviruses are very common, especially in children. However, the rotavirus vaccine will not protect against diarrhea resulting from astroviruses, caliciviruses or the many other possible causes. It is only designed to protect against a limited number of rotaviruses.[24]

Are rotavirus vaccines necessary?

Some people don't think the rotavirus vaccine is necessary. For example, one mother wrote the following:

> *"They gave my son a new vaccine for diarrhea. Are you kidding me? They injected my 2-month-old to prevent him from getting diarrhea? I was livid. And, of course, they told me that he might have diarrhea for the next 5-7 days! Can you believe that? I could've refused the shot and only risked a possibility of diarrhea instead of injecting him with something that will surely give it to him."*[25]
> —**Irate mother of a child vaccinated against rotavirus**

In developed regions of the world, like the U.S. and Europe, most cases of rotavirus are mild enough that parents can care for their babies at home. In poorer countries where diarrhea is the leading cause of child mortality, oral rehydration therapy (ORT) has proved to be quite successful. Case studies in Brazil, Egypt, Mexico and the Philippines confirm that increased use of ORT coincides with significant drops in mortality. In fact, according to a recent report on reducing deaths from diarrhea, published in the *Bulletin of the World Health Organization...*

> *"With adequate political will and financial support, cost-effective interventions other than immunization can be successfully delivered by national programs."*[26]
> —**World Health Organization**

Notes

1. Merck & Co., Inc. "RotaTeq [Rotavirus Vaccine, Live, Oral, Pentavalent]." Product insert from the vaccine manufacturer (Issued: February 2006).
2. GlaxoSmithKline. "Rotarix® (Rotavirus Vaccine, Live, Oral) Oral Suspension." Product insert from the manufacturer. (Revised: April 2008.)
3. Merck & Co., Inc. "Patient information: RotaTeq." (February 2006).
4. Vesikari, T., Matson, D., Offit, P., Clark, HF., et al. "Safety and efficacy of a pentavalent human-bovine (WC3) reassortment rotavirus vaccine." *New England Journal of Medicine*

(January 5, 2006);354:23-33.

5. National Vaccine Information Center. "MedAlerts: access to the U.S. government's Vaccine Adverse Event Reporting System (VAERS)." www.medalerts.org

6. See Note 1.

7. Ibid.

8. See Note 2.

9. Ruiz-Palacios, GM, et al. "Safety and efficacy of an attenuated vaccine against severe rotavirus gastroenteritis." *NEJM* (January 5, 2006);354:11-22. See also Table 2.

10. Linker, A. "Study: GSK vaccine may increase risk of convulsion, death." *Triangle Business Journal* (Feb 15, 2008).

11. Friedland, L. "GSK's human rotavirus vaccineRotarix®: presentation to the ACIP." *GlaxoSmithKline* (June 25, 2008).

12. Fisher, BL. "FDA panel approves Rotarix safety 11-1." *Vaccine Awakening* (February 21, 2008).

13. FDA. Center for biologics evaluation and research: product approval information—STN: BL 125122 (March 14, 2008).

14. FDA. Center for biologics evaluation and research, vaccines and related biological products advisory committee meeting (February 20, 2008).

15. Parrillo, SJ. "Pediatrics, Kawasaki disease." eMedicine, WebMD (April 15, 2008).

16. Health Canada. "Summary basis of decision (SBD) Rotarix." (July 23, 2008). www.hc-sc.gc.ca

17. See Note 2.

18. See Note 10.

19. See Note 4.

20. Ibid.

21. See Note 2.

22. See Note 1.

23. Roderick, et al. *Epidemiology and Infection* 1995;114:277-288.

24. See Notes 1 and 4.

25. Thinktwice Global Vaccine Institute. Unsolicited case report by a concerned parent. www.thinktwice.com

26. Victora, CG., et al. "Reducing deaths from diarrhoea through oral rehydration therapy." *Bulletin of the World Health Organization* 2000;78(10):1246-55.

Human Papilloma Virus (HPV)

What is HPV?

Human Papilloma Virus (HPV) is a relatively common sexually transmitted disease passed on through genital contact, usually by sexual intercourse. There are more than 100 subtypes of HPV. Some forms of the virus can cause warts (papillomas), which may appear on a woman's cervix, vagina or vulva. Other forms of the virus can cause abnormal cell growth on the lining of the cervix—cervical dysplasia—that years later can turn into cancer. However, in more than 90 percent of cases the infections are harmless and go away without treatment. The body's own defense system eliminates the virus. Often, women experience no signs, symptoms or health problems.[1]

Who is most susceptible to HPV?

People who begin having sex at an early age, who have many sex partners, or who have sex with somebody who has had many partners, are at greatest risk of contracting HPV.

How prevalent and serious is cervical cancer?

Cervical cancer incidence and death rates have consistently declined over the past 30 years. In 1975, 14.8 women (per 100,000 U.S. population) contracted the disease and 5.6 (per 100,000) died from it. By 2004, these figures had fallen by more than half: an incidence rate of 7.0 and a death rate of 2.4.[2,3] These figures are even lower in women under 50 years of age: a 5.4 incidence rate and 1.3 death rate.[4] Some experts attribute this declining death rate to the widespread use of the Pap test which detects cervical abnormalities in the early stages. When detected at an early stage, invasive cervical cancer is one of the most successfully treated cancers.[5-7]

The median age of women when they are initially diagnosed with cervical cancer is 48 years.[8] About 85 percent of all new cases are in women 35 years and older. More than half of all cervical cancer deaths are in women 55 years and older. New cervical cancer cases and deaths are uncommon below the age of 35 and nearly nonexistent before the age of 20.[9,10]

Cervical cancer is not as common as other types of cancer. For example, in 2003 there were 14.4 cases of skin cancer per 100,000 population, nearly twice the rate of cervical cancer. Rates for colon cancer, lung cancer and breast cancer were even higher. In fact, women are nearly 15 times more likely to be stricken with breast cancer than with cervical cancer.[11]

Quick Facts About HPV

♦ **HPV infections are usually harmless.** They often go away without symptoms, health problems or treatment.

♦ **Cervical cancer incidence and death rates have consistently declined over the past 30 years.** Experts attribute these declines to the expanded use of the Pap test which detects cervical abnormalities in early stages.

♦ **The median age of women when initially diagnosed with cervical cancer is 48 years.** New cervical cancer cases and deaths are uncommon below the age of 35 and nearly nonexistent before the age of 20.

♦ **Cervical cancer is not as common as other types of cancer.** For example, women are nearly 15 times more likely to be stricken with breast cancer than with cervical cancer.

The HPV vaccine:

- Gardasil—designed to protect against four of the more than 100 different HPV strains. Each dose contains "virus-like particles of the major capsid protein of HPV types 6, 11, 16 and 18." Each dose also contains sodium chloride, sodium borate, L-histidine, polysorbate 80, and "approximately 225mcg of aluminum." Produced by Merck. Licensed for females in June 2006 and for males (to combat genital warts) in September 2009. Given in 3 doses.[12]

- Cervarix—designed to protect against two of the most common strains of HPV. Each dose contains L1 proteins from HPV types 16 and 18, assembled as virus-like particles prepared by recombinant DNA technology using a "Baculovirus expression system" (gene-cloning using insect matter) in *Trichoplusia ni* cells (of the cabbage looper, a worm-like insect). Each dose also contains sodium chloride and 500mcg of aluminum. Produced by GSK. Given in 3 doses.[13]

Safety

By February 2010, just 44 months after the HPV vaccine was licensed in the U.S., more than 17,500 adverse reaction reports pertaining to Gardasil were filed with the federal government—an average of 13 reports per day.[14,15] Nearly half of all reports required a doctor or emergency room visit, with hundreds of teenage girls and young women needing extended hospitalization. In the case reports submitted to the FDA, 61 deaths were described due to blood clots, heart disease and other causes. In addition, many of the vaccine recipients were stricken with serious and life-threatening disabilities, including Guillain-Barré syndrome (paralysis), seizures, convulsions, swollen limbs, chest pain, heart irregularities, kidney failure, visual disturbances, arthritis, difficulty breathing, severe rashes, persistent vomiting, miscarriages, menstrual irregularities, reproductive complications, genital warts, vaginal lesions and HPV infection—the main reason to vaccinate.[16] According to Dr. Diane Harper, director of the Gynecologic Cancer Prevention Research Group at the University of Missouri...

"The rate of serious adverse events [from Gardasil] is greater than the incidence rate of cervical cancer."[17] —**Diane Harper, MD**

Although definitive causation has not been established, it should be noted that a confidential study conducted by a major vaccine manufacturer indicated that "a fifty-fold underreporting of adverse events" is likely.[18] In other words, perhaps only 2 percent of all adverse reactions to vaccines are revealed. Thus, nearly one million teens and young women could have been hurt by Gardasil between June 2006 and February 2010.

The case reports on the following pages were taken directly from the FDA's Vaccine Adverse Event Reporting System (VAERS).[19] They are just a small sample of the potential HPV vaccine damage to our young, female members of society. (Case numbers precede report summaries.)

Efficacy

Pre-licensure studies of Gardasil: Four studies assessed the efficacy of the HPV vaccine against HPV strains 16 and 18 (which together may cause up to 70 percent of cervical cancers), as well as strains 6 and 11 (responsible for about 90 percent of genital wart cases). The vaccine manufacturer claimed 98-100 percent efficacy.[20,21] Of course, this high efficacy rate only applies to strains in the vaccine; Gardasil will not prevent infection with HPV types not contained in the vaccine. In fact, *during clinical trials of the vaccine, hundreds of women who received Gardasil contracted HPV disease.*[22,23] Furthermore, the drug maker warns women that "vaccination does not substitute for routine cervical cancer screening."[24]

Regarding the vaccine manufacturer's staggering claim of 100 percent efficacy, it is important to realize that *no actual cases of cervical cancer were prevented in any of the test subjects in any of the clinical studies of the HPV vaccine.* In fact, the FDA admits that "the study period was not long enough for cervical cancer to develop."[25] Instead, all claims for the effectiveness of this vaccine are based on an indirect analysis of efficacy.

HPV Vaccine: VAERS Case Reports

▸268143: A 13-year-old girl received the Gardasil vaccine and nine days later was hospitalized with "ascending weakness bilaterally, upper and lower extremities." She was diagnosed by a neurologist with Guillain-Barré syndrome.

▸276255: A 14-year-old teenager was vaccinated with Gardasil. According to her physician, she subsequently developed GBS and required hospitalization.

▸277114: A 16-year-old teenager "collapsed, experienced weakness, sensory loss in extremities, and could not walk" after receiving Gardasil.

▸277667: After receiving Gardasil, an 18-year-old female felt numbness and paralysis on the right side of her face. She was diagnosed with Bell's palsy.

▸262242: A 14-year-old girl received Gardasil, lost consciousness, fell and hit her nose on a drawer. She was taken to the hospital with a broken nose.

▸275993: A 16-year-old teenager was vaccinated with Gardasil. About 15 minutes later she felt dizzy, passed out, "hitting her face and head as she fell."

▸275915: A 19-year-old student received her third dose of Gardasil, returned to her dorm, and lost consciousness in the bathroom causing a head laceration.

▸274598: A 21-year-old female received Gardasil, fainted, hit her head on the floor and suffered a concussion. She was rushed to an emergency room.

▸277575: A 13-year-old girl received her first dose of Gardasil, complained of an upset stomach, then passed out. Her eyes rolled back in her head and she began twitching. She would not regain consciousness nor respond to verbal stimulation. 911 was called and she was transported to the hospital.

▸274941: A 15-year-old girl lost consciousness and had tonic convulsions approximately 5-10 minutes after receiving her first dose of Gardasil.

▸277788: A 16-year-old teenager received her second dose of the HPV vaccine. Three days later, she had her first seizure and was taken to the emergency room. She was admitted to the hospital that evening with a grand mal seizure.

▸277351: A 13-year-old girl received Gardasil. A few hours later her entire arm, including fingers, swelled up. She had not recovered two weeks later.

▸277813: A 16-year-old teenager received her first dose of Gardasil. Later that day, she experienced back pain, chest pain, a cardiac murmur, vertigo, nausea and difficulty breathing. She was taken to the hospital by ambulance.

▸275111: A 13-year-old girl developed blood in her stool approximately three days after receiving her second dose of Gardasil. She was admitted to the hospital where she was diagnosed with "acute kidney failure."

▸275151: A 16-year-old teenager was taken to the emergency room with juvenile rheumatoid arthritis after receiving Gardasil.

▸275250: A physician reported that his 18-year-old daughter received Gardasil. Three days later, her legs became sore and her knees and ankles began to hurt. She was unable to attend school because she could no longer walk normally, and was "walking like an old lady" with pain in her extremities.

▸277664: A physician's 23-year-old daughter had disabling joint pain and arthralgia in her knees and wrists after receiving Gardasil. The pain was causing significant disability because she could not participate in former activities.

▸277402: A 21-year-old woman received her first dose of Gardasil and experienced tightness in her throat, difficulty swallowing, shortness of breath, diarrhea and headache. She required emergency room care.

▸276349: A 21-year-old female broke out in an itchy rash on her arms, chest and neck three days after being vaccinated against HPV.

▸278066: A 24-year-old woman started itching on the buttocks after HPV vaccination. The itching spread to her abdomen and thighs.

▸276240: A 17-year-old teenager received her first dose of Gardasil. She experienced extreme nausea, diarrhea and dizziness after the injection. The young lady "was vomiting so hard that the blood vessels in her eyes broke."

▸277751: A 25-year-old woman received the HPV shot and experienced persistent vomiting for several hours, requiring emergency room care.

▸274219: A 17-year-old received Gardasil during pregnancy. An ultrasound showed that the fetus had neural tube defect (of the brain and spinal cord).

▸274942: A 19-year-old female was vaccinated with her first dose of Gardasil during pregnancy and had a spontaneous abortion two weeks later.

▸274718: A mother reported that after her 11-year-old daughter received Gardasil, her next menses was longer than usual, lasting six days (instead of three days). It was also "very heavy and had a foul odor."

▸272865: A 13-year-old girl developed vaginal hemorrhage after Gardasil.

▸274729: A 14-year-old girl experienced dizziness, anemia, and "heavy menstrual cycles" after the HPV shot. Emergency room care was required.

▸274612: A 12-year-old girl developed an ovarian cyst that ruptured ten days after receiving the first dose of Gardasil. Initially, she started vomiting for a few days and then there was significant abdominal pain.

▸276564: A 17-year-old female developed "dysfunctional uterine bleeding" after receiving the HPV vaccine.

▸276147: A 15-year-old sexually *inactive* teen developed "labia lesions" soon after receiving the HPV vaccine. This adverse reaction was reported as a "vulval disorder" and required emergency room care.

▸276165: A 16-year-old girl received her first dose of the HPV vaccine. Eleven days later, she was tested for HPV and the Pap smear results were positive for high-risk HPV. Emergency room care was required.

▸275705: A gynecologist reported that his 17-year-old patient developed "severe herpes simplex genitalis" and a "superinfection" after Gardasil. She had vulval pustules and vaginal inflammation, requiring hospitalization.

▸275392: A 23-year-old woman developed venereal warts in her rectal region within three weeks after Gardasil. She had no exposure there.

▸276236: A 24-year-old woman received her first dose of the HPV vaccine. Ten days later, she developed vaginal lesions, diagnosed as genital warts.

▸282372: A 17-year-old teenager was found unconscious (lifeless) during the evening of the same day that she received her first shot of Gardasil.

▸275438: A 19-year-old teenager collapsed and died two weeks after receiving the HPV shot. The autopsy revealed large blood clots in the heart.

Scientists presume that certain "surrogate markers" or "precancerous lesions" precede cervical cancer. HPV vaccine researchers simply compared the number of these markers in women who received the vaccine to the number of these markers in women who received the placebo.[26] The prevention of these lesions is believed to result in the prevention of cervical cancer. Again, no one actually contracted cervical cancer—not in the vaccine group or placebo group—and there is no actual proof to date that even one case of cancer has been, or will be, prevented by this vaccine.

When this vaccine was being assessed for approval, the FDA asked its panel of advisors to rule on whether Gardasil protected against HPV 16 and 18, not whether it specifically prevented cervical cancer.[27] In fact, during pre-licensure studies, *361 women who received at least one shot of Gardasil went on to develop precancerous lesions on their cervixes within 3 years*—just 14 percent fewer than in the placebo control group.[28] Scott Emerson, a professor of biostatistics at the University of Washington, sat on the FDA advisory committee. He's not convinced the vaccine is worth the billions of dollars likely to be spent on it in the coming years:

> *"I do believe that Gardasil protects against HPV 16 and 18, but the effect it will have on cervical cancer rates in this country is another question entirely. There is a leap of faith involved."*[29]
> —**Scott Emerson, PhD, FDA Advisory Committee Member**

Post-marketing efficacy data:

Gardasil is being promoted as 100 percent effective. However, this is a deceptive assessment of its true ability to protect against cervical cancer. Early studies merely showed that Gardasil is effective against just two strains of cancer-causing HPV—the ones included in the vaccine— but *researchers have identified at least 15 cancer-causing HPV strains!*[30]

In 2007, after Gardasil was licensed, the *New England Journal of Medicine* examined two studies that calculated the efficacy of the HPV vaccine against *all* potentially malignant HPV types, not just the types found in the vaccine. This would provide a more honest assessment of the vaccine's likelihood to protect against cervical cancer. In the first study—the FUTURE I trial—the vaccine was shown to be just 20 percent effective. However, when the lesion types were analyzed, it was found that the vaccine was mainly reducing the number of low-risk lesions. The vaccine had *no efficacy* against higher-grade disease.[31] In the second study—the FUTURE II trial—the vaccine was shown to be just 17 percent effective. However, when the lesion types were analyzed, it was found that the vaccine was only significant against mid-risk lesions. Once again, the vaccine had *no efficacy* against higher-grade disease.[32]

Is the vaccine effective in sexually active females?

Gardasil is approved for girls and women ages 9 to 26. However, the vaccine is not effective in females who have already been exposed to the HPV strains included in the vaccine.[33] In the United States, 24 percent of females are sexually active by age 15 years, 40 percent by age 16, and 70 percent by 18 years of age.[34] Thus, lots of young teenagers have already been exposed to one or more of the HPV strains in Gardasil. In fact, a recent study found that 12 percent of all females 10 to 29 years of age tested positive for exposure to HPV-16, and 21 percent tested positive for at least one of the four HPV types included in the vaccine.[35] This is why the American Cancer Society (ACS) does not agree with the CDC's recommendation to vaccinate older teens and young women.[36] According to Dr. George Sawaya, who analyzed the pertinent HPV studies, the benefits of the vaccine are modest and the effect is fairly small. Therefore...

"The recommendation for widespread vaccination of women after they become sexually active may need to be rethought."[37]
—**George Sawaya, MD, HPV vaccine expert**

Can the HPV vaccine *increase* the risk of developing cervical cancer?

This vaccine is not only ineffective in women who have already been exposed to HPV-16 and HPV-18, but it may actually *increase* their likelihood of developing cervical cancer. When the FDA analyzed the clinical studies that the manufacturer submitted for review in its application for a license to market Gardasil, one of its main concerns was "the potential for Gardasil to *enhance* cervical disease in subjects who had evidence of persistent infection with vaccine-relevant HPV types prior to vaccination."[38] In other words, women who are already infected with low-level HPV disease (strains 6,11,16 or 18) *before* they are vaccinated with Gardasil, are likely to have their infections exacerbated by the shot. In fact, the vaccine may cause relatively harmless infections to develop into more severe, higher-grade disease. In one study of women who tested positive for "vaccine-relevant HPV" prior to receiving Gardasil, the vaccine had an efficacy of negative 45 percent (-45%). These women were significantly *more likely* (than women in the placebo group) to develop high-grade markers for cervical cancer.[39] In a gross understatement, the FDA concluded that "there is compelling evidence that the vaccine lacks therapeutic efficacy among women who have had prior exposure to HPV and have not cleared previous infection."[40]

Is the HPV vaccine causing "minor" HPV strains to flourish?

Research has shown that when vaccines only target a small number of strains capable of causing disease, less prevalent strains can replace the targeted vaccine strains. These less prevalent strains graduate from minor factors to major influences and may even become more dangerous. Scientists are now concerned that Gardasil—which only targets two of at least 15 different cancer-causing HPV strains—might be allowing HPV strains previously considered minor to flourish and become major influences. For example, in HPV vaccine study subjects, the overall incidence of HPV disease—regardless of HPV type—continued to increase, *raising the possibility that other cancer-causing HPV types eventually filled the void created after the elimination of HPV types 16 and 18.*[41] Furthermore, an analysis of data submitted to the FDA showed a disproportionate number of cases of *higher-risk* lesions that were related to non-vaccine HPV types among vaccinated women.[42]

Is the HPV vaccine mandatory?

Shortly after the HPV vaccine was licensed for 9- to 26-year-old females, and recommended for all 11- and 12-year-old girls, the manufacturer began lobbying individual states to require this vaccine for all girls before they can enter middle school. However, the legal justification for mandating vaccines is to protect the public health from contagious diseases that are spread through *casual* contact. The human papilloma virus (HPV) is *not* spread through casual contact; it is mainly transmitted through sexual intercourse. Thus, if 11- and 12-year-old girls are compelled to receive an STD vaccine, our society will have entered a new era of medical and pharmaceutical oppression. It will be easy to rationalize mandating *any* new drug or vaccine—as long as it is shown to be "effective." Currently, Gardasil may be freely accepted or rejected in most regions of the country.

What are the alternatives to this vaccine?

Numerous studies show convincing evidence that diet and nutritional factors can prevent many types of cancer, including cervical cancer, and even eliminate precursors to this disease. Fruits and vegetables, especially, have been shown to have beneficial effects against malignancies.[43-45] Among these nutritional factors, folate, or folic acid (a member of the B vitamins) has the most impressive record. Several studies show that low folate levels increase the effect of other risk factors for cervical cancer, including that of HPV infection. Conversely, high folate levels appear to be beneficial against HPV lesions and other risk factors for cervical cancer. For example, in a recent study published in a leading journal on cancer, researchers found "evidence of a protective role of folate" with regard to pre-malignant lesions of the cervix.[46] Several studies also show that folic acid supplementation can reverse cervical lesions in patients using oral contraceptives—a known risk factor for this "pre-cancerous" condition. Patients with mild and moderate cervical lesions (CIN-1 and CIN-2) showed a full reversal of their condition in just three months following a diet rich with folic acid.[47-49] Other studies confirm these results.[50-62]

A study published in the *International Journal of Cancer* found that women who ate the least amount of tomatoes had nearly five times the risk for precancerous lesions.[63] Another study measured and compared micronutrient levels in the blood of women with cervical cancer to micronutrient levels in the blood of non-cancerous women. The women with higher levels of lycopene (found in tomatoes) and vitamin A consumed greater amounts of food with these substances and had one-third less chance of developing cervical cancer.[64] Another study, published in the *American Journal of Epidemiology,* concluded that low vitamin C intake is an independent contributor to higher-grade HPV lesions.[65]

Summary:

- Cervical cancer is rare in younger females. Older women—*not* preteen and teenage girls—are most at risk for cervical cancer.
- Many of the women who develop cervical cancer did not have a Pap test. The Pap test detects cervical abnormalities in the early stages. When detected at an early stage, cervical cancer is one of the most successfully treated cancers.
- Cervical cancer is not as common as other types of cancer.
- The HPV vaccine contains aluminum, with many known and documented health hazards.
- The FDA has already received numerous reports of serious and life-threatening adverse reactions in recipients of the HPV vaccine. These include paralysis, loss of consciousness, seizures, swollen body parts, severe rashes, heart irregularities, arthritis, and death.
- Some girls and young women developed genital warts, vaginal lesions and HPV infection after receiving the HPV vaccine.
- The vaccine may be linked to reproductive complications, including miscarriages, menstrual irregularities and birth defects.

- The vaccine's highly publicized 98-100 percent efficacy rate does *not* refer to its ability to prevent cervical cancer. The vaccine is only designed to prevent a limited number of "pre-malignant" lesions that often disappear or resolve on their own.
- The vaccine has never shown that it can actually prevent cervical cancer. It has little or no effect against high grade HPV infections.
- The vaccine is only designed to protect against 4 of the more than 100 different strains of HPV.
- The vaccine is only designed to protect against two of the more than 15 different HPV strains able to develop into cervical cancer.
- The vaccine does not directly target at least 13 strains of cancer-causing HPV, so recipients of the shot may still get cervical cancer.
- The vaccine has *no efficacy* in females who have already been infected with HPV strains included in the vaccine. In fact, these women may have a *greater risk* of developing cervical cancer.
- The vaccine might be allowing HPV strains previously considered minor to flourish and become major cancer-causing influences.
- Numerous studies show that women who make a few simple changes in their diet may be able to eliminate precursors to cervical cancer and even prevent this disease.

Notes

1. National Cancer Institute. "Vaccine protects against virus linked to half of all cervical cancers." *National Inst of Health* (Nov 26, 2002). www.cancer.gov

2. National Cancer Institute. "Cervix uteri cancer (invasive): Age adjusted SEER incidence rates by year, race and age, Table V-2." *SEER Cancer Statistics Review,* 1975-2004. National Institutes of Health. www.seer.cancer.gov

3. National Cancer Institute. "Cervix uteri cancer (invasive): Age adjusted U.S. death rates by year, race and age, Table V-3." *SEER Cancer Statistics Review,* 1975-2004. National Institutes of Health. www.seer.cancer.gov

4. See Notes 2 and 3.

5. American Cancer Society. "Key statistics about cervical cancer." www.cancer.org

6. American Cancer Society. *Cancer Facts and Figures 2007,* p. 21.

7. CDC. "Cancer—cervical cancer statistics." www.apps.nccd.cdc.gov

8. National Cancer Institute. "Median age of cancer patients at diagnosis, 2000-2004; Table I-11." *SEER Cancer Statistics Review,* 1975-2004. NIH.

9. National Cancer Institute. "Age distribution (%) of incidence cases by site, 2000-2004; Table I-10." *SEER Cancer Statistics Review,* 1975-2004. NIH.

10. National Cancer Institute. "Age distribution (%) of deaths by site, 2000-2004; Table I-12." *SEER Cancer Statistics Review,* 1975-2004. NIH.

11. CDC. "Age-adjusted invasive cancer incidence rates... United States, Females 2003; Table 1.1.1.1F. *United States Cancer Statistics: 2003 Incidence and Mortality.*

12. Merck & Co., Inc. "Gardasil [Human Papillomavirus Quadrivalent (Types 6, 11, 6, 18) Vaccine, Recombinant]." Manufacturer's product insert (2009).

13. GlaxoSmithKline Biologicals. "Cervarix, Human Papillomavirus Vaccine Types 16 and 18 (Recombinant, AS04 adjuvanted)." Manufacturer's product insert (May 2007).

14. U.S. Department of Health and Human Services. "Vaccine Adverse Event Reporting System (VAERS)." www.hhs.gov

15. National Vaccine Information Center. "MedAlerts: access to the U.S. government's Vaccine Adverse Event Reporting System (VAERS)." www.medalerts.org

16. See Notes 14 and 15.

17. Chitale, R. "CDC report stirs controversy for Merck's Gardasil vaccine: cervical cancer vaccine linked to deaths, incidents of fainting and blood clots." *ABC News* (August 19, 2009).

18. Institute of Medicine. "Vaccine safety committee proceedings." (*National Academy of Sciences:* Washington, DC, May 11, 1992):40-41.

19. See Notes 14 and 15.

20. See Note 12, Table 1.

21. Medical News Today. "Merck's HPV Vaccine in Phase III Trial 100% Effective for Two Strains Causing 70% of Cervical Cancer Cases" (Oct. 9, 2005).

22. Carreyrou, J. "Questions on efficacy cloud a cancer vaccine." *The Wall Street Journal* (Apr 16, 2007):A1+.

23. Ibid., Clinical Studies.

24. See Note 12, Precautions.

25. FDA. "FDA licenses new vaccine for prevention of cervical cancer and other diseases in females caused by human papillomavirus" (June 8, 2006).

26. See Note 12, Clinical Studies; Table 1; Table 2.

27. See Note 22.

28. Ibid.

29. Ibid.

30. FDA. "Gardasil HPV Quadrivalent Vaccine, May 18, 2006 VRBPAC Meeting." Vaccines and Related Biological Products Advisory Committee Background Document.

31. Sawaya, GF., et al. "HPV vaccination—more answers, more questions." *New England Journal of Medicine* (May 10, 2007);356:1991-93.

32. Ibid.

33. See Notes 12 and 30.

34. Abma, JC., et al. "Teenagers in the United States: sexual activity, contraceptive use, and childbearing, 2002." *Vital Health Statistics 23,* 2004:1-48.

35. Jit, M., et al. "Prevalence of HPV antibodies in young female subjects in England." *British Journal of Cancer* 2007;97:989-991.

36. See Note 22.

37. Maugh II, TH., et al. "Doubts arise about cancer vaccine: benefits of HPV shots are called 'modest'; young women, parents are urged to be cautious." *Baltimore Sun* (May 10, 2007).

38. See Note 30.

39. Ibid.

40. Ibid.

41. See Note 31.

42. See Notes 30 and 31.

43. Block, G., et al. "Fruit, vegetables, and cancer prevention: a review of the epidemiological evidence." *Nutrition and Cancer* 1992;18:1-29.

44. Steinmetz, K., et al. "A review of vegetables, fruit and cancer. I. Epidemiology." *Cancer Causes and Control* 1991; 2:325-357.

45. Steinmetz, K., et al. "A review of vegetables, fruit and cancer. II. Mechanism." *Cancer Causes and Control* 1991;2:427-442.

46. Hernandez, BY., et al. "Diet and premalignant lesions of the cervix: Evidence of

a protective role for folate, riboflavin, thiamin, and vitamin B12." *Cancer Causes and Control* (Nov. 2003);14(9):859–70.

47. Butterworth CE Jr, Hatch KD, et al. "Oral folic acid supplementation for cervical dysplasia...." *Am J Obstet Gynecol.* (March 1992);166(3):803–9.

48. Butterworth, CE, et al. "Folate deficiency and cervical dysplasia." *Journal of the American Medical Association* 1992;267:528-533.

49. Butterworth, CE Jr, Hatch, KD., et al. "Improvement in cervical dysplasia associated with folic acid therapy in users of oral contraceptives." *Am J Clin Nutr.* (January 1982); 35(1):73–82.

50. Kwanbunjan, K., Saengkar, P., et al. "Folate status of Thai women cervical dysplasia." *Asia Pac J Clin Nutr.* 2004;13(Suppl):S171.

51. Sedjo, RL., Fowler, BM., et al. "Folate, vitamin B12, and homocysteine status: Findings of no relation between human papillomavirus persistence and cervical dysplasia." *Nutrition* (June 2003);19(6):839–46.

52. Goodman, MT. , et al. "Association of methyl-enetetrahydrofolate reductase polymorphism C677T and dietary folate with the risk of cervical dysplasia." *Cancer Epidemiol Biomarkers Prev.* (Dec 2001); 10(12):1275–80.

53. Weinstein, SJ., et al. "Low serum and red blood cell folate are moderately, but nonsignificantly associated with increased risk of invasive cervical cancer in U.S. women." *J Nutr.* (July 2001);131(7):2040–8.

54. Piyathilake, CJ., et al. "Methylenetetrahydrofolate reductase (MTHFR) poly-morphism increases the risk of cervical intraepithelial neoplasia." *Anticancer Res.* (May-June 2000); 20(3A):1751–7.

55. Fowler, BM. , et al. "Hypomethylation in cervical tissue: Is there a correlation with folate status?" *Cancer Epidemiol Biomarkers Prev.* (Oct 1998);7(10): 901–906.

56. Kwasniewska, A., et al. "Folate deficiency and cervical intraepithelial neoplasia." *Eur J Gynaecol Oncol.* 1997; 18(6):526–30.

57. Zarcone, R,. Et al. "Folic acid and cervix dysplasia." *Minerva Ginecol.* (Oct 1996); 48(10):397–400.

58. Christensen, B. "Folate deficiency, cancer and congenital abnormalities. Is there a connection?" *Tidsskr Nor Laegeforen.* (January 20, 1996);116(2):250–4.

59. Childers, JM., et al. "Chemoprevention of cervical cancer with folic acid: a phase III SWOG intergroup study." *Cancer Epidem Biomark Prev* 1995; 4:155-9.

60. Grio, R., et al. "Antineoblastic activity of antioxidant vitamins: folic acid in prevention of cervical dysplasia." *Panminerva Med* (Dec 1993);35(4):193–6.

61. Potischman, N., et al. "A case-control study of serum folate levels and invasive cervical cancer." *Cancer Res.* (September 1991);51(18):4785–9.

62. Whitehead, N., et al. "Megaloblastic changes in the cervical epithelium: oral contraceptive therapy and reversal with folic acid." *JAMA* 1973;226:1421-1424.

63. Van Eenwyk, J., et al. "Dietary and serum carotenoids and cervical intra-epithelial neoplasia." *Int J Canc* 1991;48:34-38.

64. Kanetsky, PA., et al. "Dietary intake and blood levels of lycopene: association with cervical dysplasia among...black women." *Nutr Cancer* 1998;31:31-40.

65. Wassertheil-Smoller, S., et al. "Dietary vitamin C and uterine cervical dysplasia." *Am J Epidemiol* (November 1981);114(5):714–24.

Multiple Vaccines

The current schedule of CDC-recommended vaccines is so crowded that doctors administer several shots during a single office visit, often with disastrous results. Today, children receive one vaccine at birth, eight vaccines at two months of age, eight vaccines at four months of age, nine vaccines at six months of age, and twelve additional vaccines between 12 and 18 months of age.[1] *The pure and innocent baby receives 38 vaccines by the time he or she is 1½ years old!*

Parents—and doctors—often forget that vaccines are drugs. (Each one contains a unique blend of chemicals, pathogens and other foreign matter.) Imagine ingesting eight or nine drugs all at one time. That's what babies get when they visit the pediatrician. In fact, these babies are not *ingesting* the drugs; instead, the drugs are being *injected* directly into their tiny bloodstreams. How often do we, as adults, ingest (or receive by injection!) eight drugs at the same time? Would we be more surprised if we *did* or *did not* have an adverse reaction?

Which vaccines do babies get by 18 months of age?

According to the CDC, babies should get the following vaccines by the time they reach 18 months of age: up to 4 doses of the hepatitis B vaccine, 3 doses of the rotavirus vaccine, 4 DTaP shots (4 doses each of diphtheria, tetanus and pertussis—12 total doses), 4 doses of the Hib vaccine (for haemophilus influenzae type B), 4 doses of the pneumococcal vaccine (Prevnar 13), 3 doses of the polio vaccine, up to 2 doses of the flu vaccine, 2 doses of the hepatitis A vaccine, an MMR shot (for measles, mumps and rubella), and a chickenpox vaccine.[2]

Why are so many vaccines given at the same time?

Several vaccines are administered simultaneously for *convenience,* not safety. Authorities believe that parents are less likely to fully vaccinate their children if they have to make extra trips to the doctor's office. However, vaccine manufacturers are not required to test their products in all of the various combinations that they are likely to be used. For example, toddlers can receive DTaP, MMR, hepatitis A and B, Hib, pneumococcal, polio, flu, and chickenpox vaccines during a single doctor visit—even though this combination of drugs was never tested for safety (or efficacy). Some children are also taking medications for other ailments. However, the vaccines that they receive were not tested in combination with these drugs.

> ## Many Babies Receive *More* than 8 or 9 Vaccines at Once
>
> Some shot dates are variable due to "age range" flexibility built into the CDC immunization schedule. Therefore...
>
> *According to the CDC, it is permissible for babies to receive up to 13 vaccines at their 12-month or 15-month doctor visits!*[3]

In addition, *vaccines are not adjusted for the weight of the child;* a 6-pound baby receives the same dose of hepatitis B vaccine—with the same amount of aluminum and formaldehyde—as a 12-pound toddler. It is also important to note that *babies are not screened prior to vaccination* to determine which ones may be more susceptible to an adverse reaction. Yet, there is ample evidence showing that when two or more drugs are taken together, this could magnify the potential for a serious adverse reaction.

Toxic synergy:

Dr. Russell Blaylock, a brain specialist and neurosurgeon, has studied the science of "toxic synergy." He notes that when two weakly toxic pesticides are used alone, neither causes Parkinson's syndrome in experimental animals. However, when they are combined, they can cause the full-blown disease quite rapidly. He likens this to multiple vaccines administered simultaneously:

> *"Vaccinations, if too numerous and spaced too close together, act like chronic illness."*[4]
> **—Russell Blaylock, MD, neurosurgeon**

Drs. Andrew Wakefield and Stephanie Cave suggested spacing some vaccines apart (MMR, for example) to lessen the potentially excessive immunological burden on the body.[5] However, it is important to understand that this strategy will not guarantee protection against serious—or even fatal—side effects. Every "body" is different; no two people react the same. *Single vaccines administered separately can, and often do, cause adverse reactions.* Still, if vaccines must be given, common sense alone tells us that several vaccines administered together are likely to be more problematic than individual shots spaced apart over a period of time.

DTaP and MMR: 3 Vaccines per Shot

Parents should understand that DTaP and MMR are each given with a single injection *but contain three vaccines.*
- The DTaP shot contains the diphtheria, tetanus, and pertussis vaccines.
- The MMR shot contains the measles, mumps, and rubella vaccines.

As an analogy, if you pour 3 small glasses of whiskey, gin, and rum into one large bottle, you're still ingesting 3 alcoholic drinks—not just one—with all of the anticipated effects.

How common are vaccine injuries?

The general public is essentially unaware of the true number of people —mostly children—who have been permanently damaged or died after receiving several vaccines simultaneously. In 1986, Congress passed the *National Childhood Vaccine Injury Act.* The "safety" provisions of this law required the government to monitor adverse reactions to vaccines. To satisfy this requirement, the FDA and CDC jointly developed a national database—the Vaccine Adverse Event Reporting System (VAERS)—so that doctors, nurses and concerned parents can report (and research) suspected reactions to vaccines. (Parents can file a report by calling 1-800-822-7967; reports can be researched by visiting www.medalerts.org.)

VAERS became available in the 1990s and immediately showed evidence of harm. In fact, *VAERS receives more than 12,000 adverse reaction reports every year.* In 2007 and 2008 alone, more than 50,000 reports were added to the database.[6] These include emergency hospitalizations, irreversible injuries, and deaths. Still, these numbers may be grossly underreported because the FDA estimates that 90 percent of doctors do not report suspected vaccine reactions. A confidential study by Connaught Laboratories, a vaccine manufacturer, indicated that "a *fifty-fold* underreporting of adverse events" is likely.[7] Yet, even this figure may be conservative. According to Dr. David Kessler, former director of the FDA, "only about one percent of serious events [adverse drug reactions] are reported."[8] (Multiply reported vaccine reactions by 100 for a more accurate sum.)

Many of the serious adverse reactions—tens of thousands of them— occurred after receiving several vaccines simultaneously.[9] A few of these reports are listed on the following page:

Multiple Vaccines Given Simultaneously: VAERS Case Reports

▶164271: A one-month-old female received DTaP, Hib, hepatitis B and inactivated polio vaccines. Ten days later she had a seizure and was admitted to the hospital. The following day she had three more seizures. The seizures increased in frequency to more than 12 per day. After 60 days, she was diagnosed with convulsions, grand mal seizures, and mental retardation.

▶98498: A two-month-old male received DTaP, Hib and inactivated polio vaccines. Two days later he developed intestinal bleeding and was hospitalized.

▶102563: A two-month-old male received DTaP, hepatitis B, Hib, and inactivated polio vaccines. Two days later he was found lifeless and cyanotic.

▶175725: A four-month-old female received DTaP, Hib, pneumococcal and inactivated polio vaccines. The following day she went into respiratory distress. After being hospitalized for 18 days, she had not recovered.

▶253421: A one-year-old male received DTaP, Hib, hepatitis B, MMR, pneumococcal, and inactivated polio vaccines. Four weeks later he developed thrombocytopenic purpura, a serious blood disorder.

▶306571: A 15-month-old boy received DTaP, MMR, hepatitis A, pneumococcal, and chickenpox vaccines. Less than 24 hours later he had prolonged seizures requiring anti-convulsants and endotracheal intubation. Other symptoms included gastroenteritis, respiratory distress, and diarrhea. He was hospitalized for 10 days.

▶289820: A two-year old boy received DTaP, Hib, polio, hepatitis B, MMR, pneumococcal, and chickenpox vaccines. He was hospitalized for cyanosis, epilepsy, grand mal convulsions, gaze palsy, screaming, and drooling.

▶231779: A five-year-old female received DTaP, MMR and inactivated polio vaccines. The following day she developed severe seizures and irregular brain patterns, with limited ability to speak and function.

▶278268: A 12-year-old girl was vaccinated with Gardasil, hepatitis A, Hib and meningococcal. The next day, she returned to the doctor with groin pain. Five days later, she developed a headache and rash, and was hospitalized for herpes zoster and viral meningitis.

▶277385: A 13-year-old girl received Gardasil along with the hepatitis A and meningococcal vaccines. 17 days later, she was taken to the hospital with hematuria (red blood cells in the urine) and Henoch-Schonlein purpura.

▶245210: A 21-year-old male received flu, meningococcal and tetanus-diphtheria vaccines. Six weeks later, he developed Guillain-Barré syndrome, facial paralysis and blurred vision. After being hospitalized for 26 days, he had not recovered.

The following pages contain a few firsthand accounts—case reports— as told by the parents of children after they had received several vaccines at the same time.[10]

Case Reports by Parents

▶ *"My son was born premature, just three pounds, three ounces at birth. At his two-month check the nurse said he needed his shots. I argued with her but she gave him four shots. I will never forget the scream he let out. Less than 24 hours later he died—and I was accused of his death!"*

▶ *"Our beautiful daughter was born in February and died in April. On the day that she died, I had taken her to the military base hospital for her two-month checkup. The doctor told me that she was just perfect. Then the doctor said that she needed four shots. She assured me that it was completely normal and that it was better to give her all at such an early age (because she wouldn't remember the shots). That evening after feeding her, we laid her down to sleep and checked on her 45 minutes later. She was dead. I told the police, coroner and investigators that I thought it was the shots because she was perfectly fine that day before the shots. But after three weeks we finally got an answer from the autopsy that it was SIDS. To this day I believe that it was the shots and no one can convince me otherwise."*

▶ *"Our son had his first round of vaccines at two months and was hospitalized for 21 days. There, he had to have blood transfusions, many, many tests, and several other medicines to save his life. No more vaccines for him."*

▶ *"My son went in for his four-month checkup, which included six vaccines. Seventeen hours later, I found him lifeless. During those last hours, he would not eat and he was sleeping way more than usual. When he would wake up, he would let out this unnerving shrill noise. It was terrifying. The agony of knowing that this could have been prevented and that the public is not aware is unbearable. Our baby will forever be remembered in our hearts."*

▶ *"My son had 5 seizures since his last shots: DTaP, Hib and MMR. He was sick at the time. They gave him his shots anyway, telling me it didn't matter."*

▶ *"My son received EIGHT vaccines: DTaP (diphtheria, tetanus, pertussis), IPV, Hib, Hep B, Prevnar and RotaTeq. He was six months old. One week later he was inconsolable and lethargic. Another three days later he presented with seizures and suffered a significant stroke. Two-thirds of his right brain is permanently damaged. I am not sure what his future holds."*

▶ *"Our son who was healthy previous to his immunizations now has asthma, celiac disease, and autism. His symptoms began almost immediately after his series of shots at 14 months when he received DTaP, MMR, polio, chickenpox and Hib. He has chronic vomiting and diarrhea, and has regressed in his development. He lost the use of language. I ache for my husband, who hasn't heard 'Daddy' from his little boy in a year. I am infuriated at the medical establishment for what they have done to my son. They can claim that his autism was inborn, but he developed normally for the first 14 months of life!"*

> ▸ *"My son received DTaP and Prevnar. The following morning he had seven seizures. He would go ghost-white and throw out his arms. They would be rigid and jerking. He stared straight ahead and didn't breathe. He used to say mama and dada; now he only babbles. He is far behind in all areas tested."*
>
> ▸ *"My dearest son died 10 hours after receiving his fourth dose of DTaP, Hib and polio vaccines. He was 20 months old. I knew he was dead when I heard my husband wailing like an animal. I grabbed his stiff and lifeless body and screamed, 'God, No, Not My Baby! He Can't Be Dead!' I administered CPR for 15 minutes, pounded on his chest, and yelled, 'Come Back, Come Back, Come Back!' Then I heard my father say over the phone to 911, 'We've got a dead baby here.' Realization hit. I opened his eyes, and he was dead. I then hugged his stiff body and emitted sounds I didn't know any human being was capable of making. I cannot adequately express my horror, anger, and ultimate suffering. My life turned upside down in one day, and each day that goes by I look at as one day closer to death, one day closer to my baby. Why? Because they told me the benefits outweigh the risks. What does that really mean, and why are these people allowed to play God?"*

Vaccines are not appropriate for everyone. They may or may not be right for you and your family. Therefore, examine credible evidence from several reputable sources prior to making your vaccine decisions. You are entitled to—and responsible for obtaining—the facts with regard to the safety, efficacy, benefits and risks of vaccination.

Notes

1. CDC. "Recommended childhood immunization schedule for persons aged 0-6 years, United States, 2010."

2. Ibid.

3. Ibid.

4. Blaylock, R. "Vaccinations: the hidden dangers." *The Blaylock Wellness Report* (May 2004):1-9.

5. "Autism: Present Challenges, Future Needs—Why the Increased Rates?" *Government Reform Committee Hearing,* Washington, DC. (April 6, 2000.) As cited in testimony.

6. National Vaccine Information Center. "MedAlerts: access to the U.S. government's Vaccine Adverse Event Reporting System (VAERS)." www.medalerts.org

7. Institute of Medicine. "Vaccine safety committee proceedings." (*National Academy of Sciences:* Washington, DC, May 11, 1992):40-41.

8. Kessler, DA. "Introducing MEDWatch: a new approach to reporting medication and device adverse effects and product problems." *Journal of the American Medical Association* (June 2, 1993):2765.

9. See Note 6.

10. Thinktwice Global Vaccine Institute. Unsolicited case reports submitted by concerned parents. www.thinktwice.com

Aluminum in Vaccines

Several vaccines contain high amounts of aluminum. Babies receive multiple doses of these aluminum-containing shots. For example, the hepatitis B vaccine (Engerix-B) is given at birth, 2 and 6 months of age. Each dose has 250 micrograms (mcg) of aluminum. The DTaP shot (Infanrix) is given at 2, 4, 6 and 15 months. Each dose has 625mcg of aluminum. The Hib vaccine (Pedvax) is given at 2, 4 and 12 months. Each dose has 225mcg of aluminum. The pneumococcal vaccine (Prevnar 13) is given at 2, 4, 6 and 12 months. Each dose has 125mcg of aluminum. The hepatitis A vaccine (Havrix) is given at 12 and 18 months. Each dose has 250mcg of aluminum. Thus, babies that follow the CDC immunization schedule are injected with nearly 5000mcg (5mg!) of aluminum by 18 months of age (see chart).[1,2] Since some shot dates are variable, *babies may receive up to 1,475mcg of aluminum at their 12-month or 15-month checkups!*

Aluminum is neurotoxic, even in minute quantities, and has a long history of well-documented hazards.[3,4] In 1927, Dr. Victor Vaughn, a toxicologist with the University of Michigan, testified before the Federal Trade Commission that "all salts of aluminum are poisonous when injected subcutaneously or intravenously."[5] According to the American Academy of Pediatrics, "Aluminum is now being implicated as interfering with a variety of cellular and metabolic processes in the nervous system and in other tissues."[6] This has led some researchers to speculate that aluminum may be linked to autism.[7,8] Some evidence appears to support this possibility. For example, in 1997 the *New England Journal of Medicine* published data showing that premature babies injected with aluminum build up toxic levels in the blood, bones and brain, and that aluminum toxicity can lead to neurological damage, including mental handicaps at 18 months of age.[9]

More recent, unpublished research led by Canadian neuroscientist Chris Shaw shows a link between the aluminum hydroxide used in vaccines, and symptoms associated with Parkinson's, ALS (Lou Gehrig's disease), and Alzheimer's. Mice injected with this common vaccine ingredient developed statistically significant increases in memory loss, anxiety, allergic skin reactions, and nerve cell damage. According to Shaw...

"[Aluminum in vaccines] is suspicious. We weren't out there to poke holes in vaccines. But all of a sudden, we've got neuron death! Either this link is known by industry and it has never been made public, or industry was never made to do these studies. I'm not sure which is scarier."[10]
—Dr. Chris Shaw, professor, University of British Columbia

Cumulative Aluminum Exposure
by 18 Months of Age

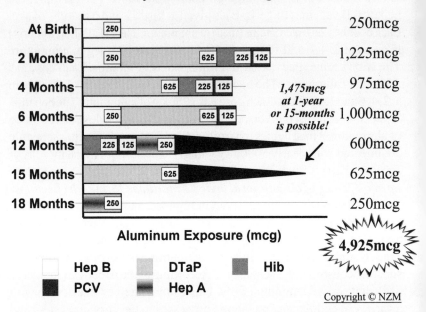

	Aluminum Exposure (mcg)	
At Birth	250	250mcg
2 Months	250 625 225 125	1,225mcg
4 Months	625 225 125	975mcg
6 Months	250 625 125	1,000mcg
12 Months	225 125 250	600mcg
15 Months	625	625mcg
18 Months	250	250mcg

1,475mcg at 1-year or 15-months is possible!

4,925mcg

Hep B   DTaP   Hib
PCV   Hep A

Babies that follow the recommended immunization schedule receive nearly 5000mcg (5mg!) of aluminum by 18 months of age. (Since some shot dates are variable, *babies may receive up to 1,475mcg of aluminum at their 12-month or 15-month checkups!*) Source: Product inserts and the CDC's immunization schedule, 2010.

Do health authorities know that aluminum is dangerous?

The Centers for Disease Control and Prevention (CDC) and the World Health Organization (WHO) are aware that aluminum is dangerous. For example, in June 2000, Dr. Tom Verstraeten, CDC epidemiologist, made the following comment to a group of concerned scientists: "The results [for aluminum] were almost identical to ethylmercury because the amount of aluminum [in vaccines] goes along almost exactly with the mercury."[11,12] He was referring to a landmark study that found "statistically significant relationships" between both aluminum and mercury in vaccines and neuro-developmental delays. Dr. John Clements, WHO vaccine advisor, provided another telling statement:

"Aluminum is not perceived, I believe, by the public as a dangerous metal. Therefore, we are in a much more comfortable wicket in terms of defending its presence in vaccines."[13] —**Dr. John Clements, WHO advisor**

The FDA is also aware that aluminum is dangerous. In a critical document on drug evaluation, the following statement is made:

> *"Research indicates that patients with impaired kidney function, including premature neonates, who receive [injections] of aluminum at greater than 4 to 5mcg per kilogram of body weight per day, accumulate aluminum at levels associated with central nervous system and bone toxicity. Tissue loading may occur at even lower rates."*[14] —**FDA document**

This means that for a 6 pound baby, 11-14mcg would be toxic. The hepatitis B vaccine given at birth contains 250mcg of aluminum—*20 times higher than safety levels!* Babies weigh about 12 pounds (5.5kg) at two months of age when they receive 1,225mcg of aluminum from their vaccines—*50 times higher than safety levels!*

Of course, healthy babies without impaired kidney function may be able to handle more aluminum. However, no one knows how much more because such studies were never conducted. In addition, babies are not screened for kidney strength prior to vaccination. Therefore, it's impossible to know ahead of time which babies will succumb to aluminum poisoning. Instead, parents are expected to play Russian Roulette with their children (see table). Aluminum-free vaccines are a safer alternative.

Notes

1. CDC. "Recommended childhood immunization schedule for persons aged 0-6 years, United States, 2010."
2. Data on aluminum content is taken directly from the manufacturers' product inserts.
3. Zatta, P., et al. "Aluminum and health." First International Conference on Metals and the Brain: from Neurochemistry to Neurodegeneration. University of Padova, Italy (Sep 20-23, 2000).
4. Wisniewski, HM., et al. "Aluminum neurotoxicity in mammals." *Environmental Geochemistry and Health* (March 1990);12(1-2):115-20.
5. Ayoub, D. "Aluminum, vaccines and autism: déjà vu!" National Autism Association Annual Conference. Atlanta, GA. (Nov. 11, 2007).
6. Committee on Nutrition. "Aluminum toxicity in infants and children." *Pediatrics* (March 1996);97(3):413-416.
7. See Note 5.
8. Taylor, G. "It's not just the mercury: aluminum hydroxide in vaccines." *Adventures in Autism* (March 9, 2008). www.adventuresinautism.blogspot.com
9. Bishop, NJ., et al. "Aluminum neurotoxicity in preterm infants receiving intravenous-feeding solutions." *NEJM* 1997; 336(22):1557-62.
10. Woolley, P. "Vaccines show sinister side." *Vancouver Free Press* (Mar 23, 2006).
11. This statement was made in June 2000 at a top-secret meeting of health officials held at the Simpsonwood conference center in Norcross, Georgia. Data accessed FOIA.
12. From transcripts of the meeting (accessed via Freedom of Information Act).
13. Clements, J. "Workshop on aluminum in vaccines." Presented by National Vaccine Program Office, Dept. of HHS. San Juan, PR (May 11-12, 2000).
14. Rappaport, B. "Doc. NDA 19-626/S-019." *FDA: Office of Drug Evaluation II, Center for Drug Eval. & Research* (Feb 13, 2004): Sec.3a. www.fda.gov/cder/foi/appletter

Vaccines that Contain Aluminum

Some vaccines contain aluminum salts, which are added as adjuvants to help the vaccine stimulate a better response and increase efficacy. There are three types of aluminum-containing adjuvants used in vaccines: 1) aluminum hydroxide, also referred to as aluminum hydroxyphosphate sulfate (AH), 2) aluminum phosphate (AP), and 3) aluminum potassium sulfate (APS). The following vaccines contain aluminum:

Vaccine	Product Name	Aluminum per Dose
Polio (IPV)	Pediarix (IPV, DTaP, Hep B)	850mcg (AH,AP)
	Pentacel (IPV, DTaP, Hib)	1500mcg* (AP)
	Quadracel (IPV, DTaP)	1500mcg* (AP)
DTaP	Pediarix (DTaP, Hep B, IPV)	850mcg (AH,AP)
	Pentacel (DTaP, IPV, Hib)	1500mcg* (AP)
	Quadracel (DTaP, IPV)	1500mcg* (AP)
	TriHIBit (DTaP, Hib)	170mcg (APS)
	Daptacel (DTaP)	1500mcg* (AP)
	Tripedia (DTaP)	170mcg (APS)
	Infanrix (DTaP)	625mcg (AH)
	Boostrix (Tdap)	390mcg (AH)
	Adacel (Tdap)	1500mcg* (AP)
Tetanus/DT/Td	Tetanus/S. Pasteur (TT)	250mcg (APS)
	Tet-Dip/S. Pasteur (DT)	170mcg (APS)
	Decavac (Td)	280mcg (APS)
HPV	Gardasil	225mcg (AH)
	Cervarix	500mcg (AH)
Hepatitis A	Vaqta (Hep A)	225/450mcg–child/adult (AH)
	Havrix (Hep A)	250/500mcg–child/adult (AH)
	Twinrix (Hep A & B)	450mcg (AH,AP)
Hepatitis B	Pediarix (HepB, DTaP, IPV)	850mcg (AH,AP)
	Comvax (Hep B, Hib)	225mcg (AH)
	Twinrix (Hep A & B)	450mcg (AH,AP)
	Recombivax (Hep B)	250/500mcg–child/adult (AH)
	Engerix-B (Hep B)	250/500mcg–child/adult (AH)
Hib	Pentacel (Hib, DTaP, IPV)	1500mcg* (AP)
	TriHIBit (Hib, DTaP)	170mcg (APS)
	Comvax (Hib, Hep B)	225mcg (AH)
	PedvaxHib (Hib)	225mcg (AH)
Pneumococcal	Prevnar 13	125mcg (AP)

*According to the manufacturer, each dose contains:
"1500mcg aluminum phosphate (330mcg of aluminum) as the adjuvant."

Source: The vaccine manufacturers' product inserts. (Note: This list is intended as a general guide and does not include all vaccines that may contain aluminum. For accurate, up-to-date information, contact the individual manufacturers.)

Ingredients in Vaccines

Parents should understand that vaccines are drugs. They contain antigens, preservatives, adjuvants, stabilizers, antibiotics, buffers, diluents, emulsifiers, excipients, residuals, solvents, and inactivating chemicals.[1,2] They also contain residue from animal and human growth mediums. Here is a partial list of vaccine ingredients, with brief comments:

ANTIGENS: The main component of any vaccine, designed to induce an immune response. These are either weakened germs or fragments of the disease organism: **viruses** (*polio*), **bacteria** (*Bordetella pertussis*), and **toxoids** (*Clostridium tetani*) are examples.

GROWTH MEDIUMS: Viruses require a medium in which to propagate. Common broths include chick embryo fibroblasts; chick kidney cells; mouse brains; African green monkey kidney (Vero) cells; and human diploid (fetal) cells (MRC-5, RA 27/3, WI-38).

PRESERVATIVES: Are used to stop microbial contamination of vaccines. **Thimerosal (mercury)** is a recognized developmental toxin and suspected immune, kidney, skin and sense organ toxin. **Benzethonium chloride** is a suspected endocrine, skin and sense organ toxin. **2-phenoxyethanol** is a suspected developmental and reproductive toxin; chemically similar to antifreeze. **Phenol** is a suspected blood, developmental, liver, kidney, neuro, reproductive, respiratory, skin and sense organ toxin.

ADJUVANTS: Are used to enhance immunity. **Aluminum salts** are the most common. There is some evidence that **squalene** may have been added to anthrax vaccines, and may be linked to Gulf War illnesses. It has also been added to some recent, experimental swine flu vaccines.

STABILIZERS: Inhibit chemical reactions and prevent vaccine contents from separating or sticking to the vial. **Fetal bovine (calf) serum** is a commonly used stabilizer. **Monosodium glutamate (MSG)** helps the vaccine remain unchanged when exposed to heat, light, acidity, or humidity. **Human serum albumin** helps stabilize live viruses. **Porcine (pig) gelatin,** which protects vaccines from freeze-drying or heat, can cause severe allergic reactions.

ANTIBIOTICS: Prevent bacterial growth during vaccine production and storage. **Neomycin** is a developmental toxin and suspected neurotoxin. **Streptomycin** is a suspected blood, skin and sense organ toxin. **Polymyxin B** is a suspected liver and kidney toxin.

ADDITIVES (Buffers, diluents, emulsifiers, excipients, residuals, solvents, etc.): Some of these, such as **sodium chloride**, are probably benign. **Egg proteins** and **yeast** can cause severe reactions. **Ammonium sulfate** is a suspected liver, neuro and respiratory toxin. **Glycerin** is a suspected blood, liver and neuro toxin. **Sodium borate** is a suspected blood, endocrine, liver and neuro toxin. **Polysorbate 80** (Tween 80) is a suspected skin and sense organ toxin. **Hydrochloric acid** is a suspected liver, immune, locomotor, respiratory, skin and sense organ toxin. **Sodium hydroxide** is a suspected respiratory, skin and sense organ toxin. **Potassium chloride** is a suspected blood, liver and respiratory toxin.

INACTIVATING CHEMICALS: These kill unwanted viruses and bacteria that could contaminate vaccines. **Formaldehyde** (or **formalin**) is a known carcinogen and suspected liver, immune, neuro, reproductive, respiratory, skin and sense organ toxin; used in embalming fluids. **Glutaraldehyde** is a suspected developmental, immune, reproductive, respiratory, skin and sense organ toxin. **Polyoxyethylene** is a suspected endocrine toxin.

CONTAMINANTS: Vaccines may also contain dangerous, unintended substances, such as SV-40 found in some polio vaccines, and HIV discovered in early hepatitis B vaccines.

Notes

1. The vaccine manufacturers' product inserts.
2. Chemical profiles: www.scorecard.org

Social Obligation

Do parents have a social obligation to vaccinate their children?
Health officials often claim that parents have an obligation to vaccinate their children. They say that vaccines won't work for society unless a high percentage of children are injected. Apparently, unvaccinated children are a threat to the group. But this does not make sense. By this reasoning, the unvaccinated—who are being coerced into taking the shots—*are somehow responsible for protecting the vaccinated.* How ironic!

If some children are vaccinated, that's their family's choice. If other children are unvaccinated, that's their family's informed decision as well. Vaccinated children take their chances hoping to avoid serious adverse reactions, while unvaccinated children risk contracting the disease. However, *if vaccinated children contract the disease, the shot was ineffective, NOT the fault of unvaccinated children.* Officials ignore their own ineffective vaccine, choosing instead to malign the unvaccinated. Outrage should be vented in the proper direction—at those who developed ineffective shots and falsely promoted a defective product.

Health officials respond to this argument by claiming that some people have weak immune systems and therefore cannot take certain vaccines. Thus, your child should be vaccinated to protect these frail members of society. However, vaccine manufacturers actually warn recently vaccinated children to stay away from people with compromised immune systems because the vaccine virus could spread and cause serious complications.[1] When vaccinated children spread disease to other people, authorities euphemistically call these new cases "secondary transmissions." They are well documented in the medical literature.

Should parents be obligated to play Russian Roulette?
Vaccines pose serious risks. These hazards are acknowledged by vaccine manufacturers in their product inserts, documented in numerous studies, substantiated by the federal government's Vaccine Adverse Event Reporting System (VAERS), and confirmed anecdotally by parents. For example, the MMR vaccine manufacturer concedes that diabetes, thrombocytopenia (a serious blood disorder), arthritis, encephalitis (brain inflammation), Guillain-Barré syndrome (paralysis), and death, have all been reported during clinical trials of its vaccine. Important studies link the haemophilus influenzae type b (Hib) vaccine to epidemics of type 1 diabetes, the hepatitis B vaccine to autoimmune and neurological disorders (including multiple

sclerosis), and the flu vaccine to paralytic disability. These are just a few examples. Medical and scientific journals contain hundreds of other peer-reviewed studies linking vaccines to debilitating ailments.

In addition, every year approximately 15,000 people file vaccine adverse reaction reports with the CDC. Many of these cases are serious, requiring hospitalization, resulting in life-threatening disabilities, or death. VAERS is a *passive* reporting system, so the number of people believed to be hurt by vaccines is vastly underreported. According to Dr. David Kessler, former head of the FDA, "only about 1 percent of serious events—adverse drug reactions—are reported."[2] This is confirmed by the unsolicited personal stories that I hear about all the time. The families telling these dreadful stories rarely file official reports. Of course, these stories do not constitute "proof" of vaccine damage—at least no more than a child's cry after skinning his knee is "proof" of pain. However, patterns of adverse vaccine reactions are easily observed when unrelated families consistently report similar stories of healthy children prior to their shots, and hospitalized children after their shots. These patterns tell a larger story.

A vaccine industry that errs on the side of denial rather than concern is backward and negligent. In an enlightened healthcare community, we would listen to the larger story with sincerity and opt to protect additional children from harm. Pretending that serious reactions to vaccines are rare does not make it true, incapacitates our children, and degrades our society. Since reputed vaccine risk-to-benefit ratios are spurious, and "preventive" shots are markedly more unsafe than officially acknowledged, *it is morally unconscionable to mandate vaccines for children.*

Some recommended vaccines are clearly unnecessary:

Our children have become captive instruments of the vaccine industry, accessible by mandate. For example, children rarely develop hepatitis B. In the United States, less than 1% of all reported hepatitis B cases occur in persons less than 15 years of age. When the hepatitis B vaccine was initially introduced, 87% of pediatricians did NOT believe it was needed by their patients. Doctors knew that children *rarely* develop this disease. According to the hepatitis B vaccine manufacturer, children are targeted "because a vaccination strategy limited to high-risk individuals has failed."[3] In other words, because high-risk groups—sexually promiscuous adults and IV drug users—are difficult to reach or have rejected this vaccine, authorities are targeting children. Authorities believe that by vaccinating children (a low-risk *herd*) they will protect unvaccinated adults (a high-risk *herd*). Since children are unlikely to catch hepatitis B, and studies show that vaccine efficacy declines after a few years, *children are being subjected to all of the risks of the hepatitis B vaccine without the expected benefit.*

The chickenpox vaccine is another drug that should not have been mandated for all children. It was available since the 1970s but authorities were reluctant to license and promote it because the disease is rarely dangerous and confers lifelong immunity. The vaccine, however, contains a weakened form of the virus; once injected, it remains in the body indefinitely. Authorities were concerned that it could reawaken years after the vaccination and cause serious problems. In addition, the chickenpox vaccine was originally developed for children with leukemia or compromised immune systems, a small population at greater risk for complications from the disease. But vaccine manufacturers quickly sought a wider market for their potentially lucrative product. A study conducted by the CDC in 1985 determined that the vaccine was not necessary. However, in 1995 it was promoted as "cost-effective"—rather than essential—because moms and dads would not have to miss work and stay home (an average of 1 day) to care for their sick children. It was licensed shortly thereafter.

Before the chickenpox vaccine was licensed, doctors would encourage parents to expose their children to the disease while they were young. Doctors recommended this course of action because they knew that chickenpox is relatively harmless when contracted prior to the teenage years (but more dangerous in adolescents and adults). However, *after* the vaccine was licensed, the CDC began warning parents about the dangers of chickenpox. Doctors stopped encouraging parents to expose their children to this disease. Instead, they were told to have their children vaccinated.

These examples confirm that some recommended vaccines are NOT essential. Low-risk children are being force-vaccinated to protect high-risk adults or to increase the vaccine manufacturer's profits. Therefore, *requiring parents to vaccinate their children, or threatening to withhold a child's education for refusing needless vaccines, is a moral outrage.*

Conflicts of interest permeate the vaccine industry:

Vaccine recommendations and other important healthcare decisions that affect our nation's children are frequently based on ulterior motives. Safety and protection are NOT always top priorities. Instead, authorities may be influenced by monetary considerations or the urge to manipulate undesirable study results. For example, in June of 2000, two separate yet highly significant events rocked the vaccine industry:

Event #1: Congress held a hearing to determine if "the entire process [of licensing and recommending vaccines] has been polluted and the public trust has been violated."[4] Two years earlier, vaccine authorities had evidence that a new vaccine under consideration (for diarrhea!) was dangerous, yet that didn't stop them from licensing and recommending it for every child in the USA. This vaccine was linked to numerous cases of a life-threatening intestinal blockage and baby deaths. After this vaccine was withdrawn from the market, Congress discovered that 60 percent of the FDA advisory committee members who voted to license this defective vaccine, and 50 percent of the CDC advisory committee members who voted to recommend it for every child in the country, had financial ties to the drug company that produced the vaccine or to two other companies developing their own potentially lucrative competing vaccines.[5] Despite this important Congressional exposé, no one at the FDA, CDC, or U.S. Department of Health and Human Services admitted a problem, and claimed that it's perfectly acceptable for committee members with obvious conflicts of interest to make healthcare recommendations for every child in the USA—even when they stand to benefit financially from their own decisions!

Event #2: Just one week prior to the Congressional investigation into conflicts of interest within the vaccine industry, a top-secret meeting of high-level officials from the CDC, FDA, World Health Organization (WHO), and representatives from every major vaccine manufacturer, was held at the secluded Simpsonwood conference center in Norcross, Georgia. They had gathered to discuss an alarming new study that *confirmed a link between thimerosal (mercury) in childhood vaccines and neurological damage,* including recent dramatic increases in autistic spectrum disorders. However, instead of warning the public and recalling the dangerous vaccines, this small group of federal health officials and vaccine industry executives spent the weekend calculating how to cover up the truth—and followed through on their plot over the next few years. (This story was discussed in greater detail in the chapter on autism.)

These two events—the Congressional hearing on conflicts of interest within the vaccine licensing and recommendation process, and the secret Simpsonwood conference—confirm that U.S. health authorities have lost their ethical bearings and have NOT made our children's safety a top priority. Requiring parents to vaccinate their children when the shots may have been added to the immunization schedule simply to line the pockets of powerful authorities is dangerous and corrupt. Withholding a child's education for refusing vaccines when crucial studies purporting to prove their safety are bogus, is both reprehensible and indefensible. Thus, *every family must remain free to accept or reject vaccines.*

Are vaccines mandatory?

Manufacturers produce vaccines for the FDA to license and regulate. The CDC establishes a recommended schedule. State legislators then write the laws dictating who must be vaccinated within their state (usually children) and how often. Schools and other institutions enforce the laws. However, vaccines are not legally required under several circumstances.

Young children: Babies born at hospitals may be subjected to a hepatitis B vaccine within hours of birth. However, this is a hospital policy, not a state law. Parents can withhold consent. (If parents reject the shot, they must never let the baby out of eyesight at the hospital because personnel have been known to vaccinate newborns against the parents' wishes.)

Children taken to the doctor for well-baby visits are expected to receive several vaccines. However, these are merely recommended by the CDC and encouraged by the pediatrician. Unless the state you live in mandates these vaccines for infants, they are not legally required. If you object to the shots, your doctor may lecture and frighten you with horror stories about unvaccinated children contracting diseases and dying. Some doctors challenge the parents' competence or even threaten to call Social Services for child neglect. Many abandon their patients, refusing to see them again. Parents should be thankful that this dysfunctional relationship with their health care practitioner has been terminated. Naturopathic doctors are an option and can be found in the local telephone book.

Public school: State vaccine laws are generally written to regulate enrollment in public institutions. Vaccines may be required to enter daycare, public school or college. However, all states offer legal exemptions to "mandatory" vaccines. If you do not wish to vaccinate your child but would still like to enroll your child in a public school, acquire a copy of your state vaccine law to determine which exemptions are permitted.

All states permit a **medical exemption** if a doctor will certify that vaccines might hurt the child. (Doctors rarely provide a medical waiver. When they do, it's usually to exempt just one or two vaccines.)

Most states offer a **religious exemption**, but each state has a different way of defining it. Again, acquire a copy of your state vaccine law to determine precise requirements. (Contrary to popular belief, religious exemptions do not have to be written by the head of a church.)

Some states also offer a **philosophical exemption**. For example, Arizona, California, and Colorado allow parents to enroll their children in public school without vaccines if they sign a letter indicating that they have "beliefs" opposed to vaccines. The law does not require parents to elaborate upon their beliefs. Several other states also permit philosophical exemptions. Simply sign the vaccine waiver and submit it. Authorities are legally obligated to honor the exemption.

Private institution: Private schools, clubs, camps, daycares, and colleges are not obligated to honor religious or philosophical exemptions, although many choose to accept non-vaccinated students. Be sure to call the private institution prior to beginning the application process to ascertain their vaccine policy. Otherwise, your child may be removed from the institution after he or she has been enrolled.

Make an informed vaccine decision:

The eminent pediatrician, Dr. Robert Mendelsohn, promoted vaccines until he realized they were harming his patients. He stopped recommending vaccines and started speaking out against them. Like Dr. Mendelsohn, I am convinced that vaccines do more harm than good. However, *you* must decide whether they are appropriate for your family. If you choose not to vaccinate, there are risks involved. Your child could contract a disease for which a vaccine has been developed. Your child could even die. On the other hand, by not vaccinating you will avoid the unpredictable dangers associated with recommended shots.

Please visit my website at www.homefirst.com for more information, or visit www.thinktwice.com for additional resources. I also sincerely recommend that you balance the information presented in this book with official information from your health practitioner, vaccine manufacturers, the FDA, CDC, and World Health Organization. You will then be ready to *Make an Informed Vaccine Decision for the Health of Your Child*.

Notes

1. See product inserts for MMR, chickenpox and rotavirus.
2. Kessler, DA. "Introducing MEDWatch: a new approach to reporting medication and device adverse effects and product problems." *JAMA* (June 2, 1993):2765.
3. See product insert for hepatitis B vaccine.
4. "Conflicts of Interest and Vaccine Development: Preserving the Integrity of the Process." *Govt. Reform Committee Hearing,* Washington, DC. (June 15, 2000.) As cited in Chairman Dan Burton's opening statement.
5. "Conflicts of Interest in Vaccine Policy Making Majority Staff Report." *Committee on Government Reform,* U.S. House of Representatives (June 15, 2000). As cited in section IV, FDA, VRBPAC; B. Conflict of Interest Review and Waivers by the FDA.

Index

222 Make an Informed Vaccine Decision

About the Authors

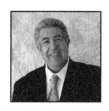

Mayer Eisenstein, MD, JD, MPH is a graduate of the University of Illinois Medical School, the Medical College of Wisconsin School of Public Health, and the John Marshall Law School. He is Board Certified by the National Board of Medical Examiners, American Board of Public Health and Preventive Medicine, and the American Board of Quality Assurance and Utilization Review Physicians. He is a recipient of the Howard Fellowship, Health Professional Scholarship, University of Illinois School of Medicine Scholarship, and is a member of the Illinois Bar.

Dr. Mayer Eisenstein is the Medical Director of Homefirst® Health Services, the largest physician and midwife attended homebirth practice in the United States. Homefirst provides a full range of family healthcare services in the greater Chicago metropolitan area, with four medical centers. Since 1973, Homefirst doctors have delivered over 15,000 babies at home —most of whom have never been vaccinated—serving more than 75,000 parents, grandparents, and children.

Dr. Eisenstein has practiced medicine, delivered babies, and provided families with preventive healthcare services for over 35 years. Since 1987, his weekly call-in radio program, *The Doctor and the Pharmacist,* has aired in Chicago. Some of his guest appearances on television include *Phil Donahue, Hannity and Colmes,* and *Oprah Winfrey.* In addition, he is the author of *The Home Birth Advantage* and *Unlocking Nature's Pharmacy.* Dr. Eisenstein's healthcare philosophy—minimal reliance upon prescription drugs, antibiotics, and medical intervention as a first line of treatment—comes from his many years in medicine, public health, and law, combined with his years as a husband, father, and grandfather.

Homefirst® Health Services
www.homefirst.com

Neil Z. Miller is a medical research journalist and the Director of the *Thinktwice Global Vaccine Institute.* He is the author of several books and articles on vaccines, including *Vaccine Safety Manual for Concerned Families and Health Practitioners* and *Vaccines: Are They Really Safe and Effective?* Mr. Miller is a frequent guest on radio and TV talk shows, including *PBS, Phil Donahue,* and *Montel Williams.* Mr. Miller has a degree in psychology and is a member of Mensa. He lives in Northern New Mexico with his family.

Thinktwice Global Vaccine Institute
www.thinktwice.com

Purchasing Information

Additional copies of this book, **Make an Informed Vaccine Decision** (ISBN: 978-188121736-7), may be purchased directly from *New Atlantean Press*. Call 505-983-1856. Or send $14.95 (in U.S. funds), plus $5.00 shipping, to:

New Atlantean Press
PO Box 9638
Santa Fe, NM 87504
505-983-1856 (Telephone & Fax)
Email: think@thinktwice.com

This book is also available at many fine bookstores and health stores.

Bookstores/Libraries/Retail Buyers: Order from Midpoint, Baker &Taylor, Ingram, New Leaf, Nutri-Books, or New Atlantean Press. In Europe, contact Gazelle; in Australia and New Zealand, this book is distributed by Brumby Books.

Chiropractors and other Non-Storefront Buyers: Take a 40% discount with the purchase of 5 or more copies (multiply the total cost of purchases x .60). Please add 9% ($5.00 minimum) for shipping. *Larger discounts are available.*

Shipping Rates

United States (1 or 2 books): Please add $5.00 for media mail (allow 1-2 weeks for your order to arrive) or include $2.00 extra ($7.00 total) for Priority shipping.
Canada and Mexico: Please add $12.00 for Global Priority shipping.
Europe, Asia and Australia: Please add $14.00 for Global Priority shipping.

More Vaccine Resources

VACCINE SAFETY MANUAL (2nd Edition) for Concerned Families and Health Practitioners (ISBN: 978-188121737-4). The world's most complete guide to immunization risks and protection. Includes more than 1,000 scientific citations. More than 100 charts, graphs and illustrations supplement the text. This encyclopedic health manual is an important addition to every family's home library and will be referred to again and again. Code: VSM (352pages) $19.95.

Vaccines: Are They *Really* Safe and Effective? (ISBN: 978-188121730-5). An excellent introductory book on vaccine safety and efficacy issues. Includes 30 charts and more than 900 citations. Code: VAC (128 pages) $12.95.

Vaccine Guide for Dogs and Cats (ISBN: 1-88121734-5). An important resource that includes hundreds of studies to help pet lovers make informed and responsible decisions. Code: ANI (128 pages) $13.95.

ONLINE CATALOG

New Atlantean Press offers many excellent publications on vaccines, holistic health, natural parenting, and conscious childcare. We also offer several top-of-the-line holistic products, including gifts for women, homeopathic kits, and more. For more information, visit: www.thinkchoice.com